# MODERN HAIR RESTORATION

## A Complete Hair Loss Guide
### For Men and Women
### 3rd Edition

## by
## Parsa Mohebi, MD

MODERN HAIR RESTORATION
A Complete Hair Loss Guide For Men and Women
3rd Edition

# Contents

I

III

IV

***Dedicated to my patients,**
For their trust and the gift of achievement
they give me every day.
I respect them for choosing to transform their lives*

# INTRODUCTION

## HAIR AND IMAGE

*"The self-image is the key to human personality and human behavior. Change the self-image and you change the personality and the behavior."*
**Maxwell Maltz**, *(1899-1975)*

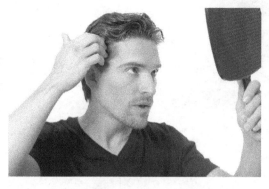

Self-image is important to us and hair plays a significant role in the way we view ourselves. By the age of fifty, over fifty percent of American men will experience some degree of hair loss that may require medical attention. Although it was thought to be a strictly male disease, women

---

1. Maltz, Maxwell (1899-1975) was a cosmetic surgeon who developed Psycho Cybernetics, a system of ideas that can be employed to improve one's self-image and in turn lead a more successful and fulfilling life.

actually make up a large number of American hair loss sufferers. Hair loss in women is often devastating for their self-image and emotional well-being. As a medical doctor specializing in hair restoration, other physicians and I often hear comments such as:

> *"I don't feel good about myself since I started losing my hair."*

> *"I always feel a bit down since my hair started falling out."*

> *"I hate the way I look, some guys are lucky with the bald look, I'm not one of them."*

> *"I look just like my father now; too bad I'm only 28 years old."*

Our self-image is a multi-dimension of complexity in which we see and interpret ourselves. Self-image is the internal unseen thoughts that frame us and how we perceive our physical appearance and how we value it. Our physical appearance contributes greatly to our self-image. In our quiet internal dialogue, most people ponder on how the world sees them and a good portion of our life is spent working on what we present to the world. Our hair is one of the physical features that reflects how we perceive and feel about ourselves on many levels.

Of course, we are more than the sum total of our physical appearance. Still, we live for the most part in a seeing world and what we see provides great sensory awareness. What we see shapes our sense of what we find appealing. This is true of our own self-imaging. Like it or not; hair plays a significant role in our self- image.

In ancient Egypt, men generally kept their hair short or shaved it off and wealthy Egyptian men wore wigs. The women kept their hair long, plaited and curled. The wealthy women also wore elaborate wigs. During the 1000 years of heightened Egyptian civilization, hair fashion was intricate to social status, the priesthood and the God-like status of the Pharaohs.

Our hair and face are the single most defining physical attributes of our self-image. When a person begins losing hair, his/her self-esteem is often lost with it. Having healthy, shiny, brilliant hair is equated to power, beauty, sexiness and success. This underscores why people's self-esteem levels drop significantly when hair loss occurs. This long-standing social phenomenon makes hair loss a negative event for both men and women.

The Internal Revenue Service (IRS) noted, in 2001, that the American hair industry generated 25.3-billion dollars on haircuts, styling, coloring and more. This simple keratinized protein we call hair is a major sector of our economics and a major factor in a positive personal self-image.

Women are known for spending a lot of time and money grooming, dying, curling, drying and styling their hair to make it look its best. When they begin to lose their hair, it can be an extremely traumatic experience. Even though in the urban metro sexual era, men do a good share of this, the cosmetic setback is quite intense when a woman is used to

2. 2001, Cash Intensive Businesses Audit Techniques Guide - Chapter 10; http://www.irs.gov/businesses/small/article/0,,id=210745,00.html

having hair and suddenly finds herself losing it. They can have a lot of trouble dealing with the reality of hair loss.

Self-esteem in men is also significantly affected by hair loss. Hair loss causes both men and women to look older and this is what worries many people. The aging factor is a large part of the reason people lose their self-esteem when they lose their hair. Emotional problems that come from hair loss can interfere with every aspect of someone's life including love, career and relationships. The stress that comes with hair loss only worsens the situation.

If you experience hair loss and it is affecting your life, the best thing to do is determine the cause of the hair loss and visit a qualified physician for a consultation to discuss hair restoration treatment options.

## PSYCHOLOGICAL IMPACTS OF BALDING

Balding, and its psychological impact, has been the subject of many studies in the past. The relationship between hair loss and stress is clear to all clinicians who practice in this field. Negative psycho social impacts of hair loss in male patterned baldness and in women with hair thinning or balding have also been seen. Many hair transplant surgeons observe the negative effects of hair loss on self-esteem and self-image in their patients.

Reported effects from some male patients include:
- Detrimental impact on their sex life
- Affected career choices in men
- Inability to stay competitive in the workplace

- Increased anxiety levels among younger men
- A higher rate of depression in men with male patterned baldness

There has been solid evidence and published literature on the psychological impacts of hair loss in both men and women. However, the corrective effect of medical and surgical hair restoration has not been studied until recently. After observing the drastic changes in patient's behavior and the high level of patient satisfaction in those who have had a hair transplant, we were motivated to look into the psychological impact of hair restoration on different aspects of a patient's life.

## A UNIQUE STUDY ON THE PSYCHOLOGICAL EFFECTS OF HAIR LOSS

In 2008, Dr. William Rassman and I conducted a unique study to quantify the psycho social impact of hair loss in men with typical male patterned baldness. We came up with a series of criteria based on previous studies and our clinical observations that could have been modified by having a hair restoration procedure. We utilized indices that were previously studied comparing bald and non-bald men on different psychological variables.

Initially, a pilot study was performed in which patients were asked about different aspects of their lives during their post-op visits. Patients received open ended questionnaires eliciting responses as to their psychological state after their hair restoration procedure was completed. Based on the pilot study, we focused on eight major criteria reported and documented as variables associated with hair loss in the literature.

A subset of patients from our pilot study was collected. These questionnaires included questions on their general level of happiness, energy level, feeling of youthfulness, anxiety levels, self-confidence, outlook on their future and even the impact on their career and sex life. We chose patients who had their first hair transplant surgery one to three years prior to the time of the study. This meant the patients had clearly experienced the results of their hair restoration procedure. This study was limited to men with male patterned baldness. It was anticipated that patients whose surgeries were less than three years back would have strong memory recall. The patients chosen had received follicular unit transplants that reflected the best standard of care in hair restoration.

Two hundred questionnaires were sent to this group of hair transplant recipients. It also included a brief description on the nature of the scientific study. Patients were permitted to respond anonymously and their participation was voluntary. We found out that the patients had significant improvements in all eight criteria regardless of their stage of baldness and their ages. In the graph below, Figure 1 shows that, in 18% of the respondent group, there was a greater sense of wellbeing in their overall happiness, energy levels, careers, sex life and youthfulness. Respondents also felt a sense of decreased anxiety, improvement in self-confidence and outlook on life.

Our study confirms the significance of hair to people's self-image and esteem.

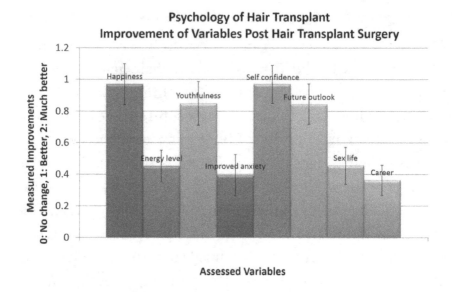

*Figure 1: Illustrates the improvement of psycho social variables quantified in the Mohebi/Rassman Study of hair restoration patients in 2008.*

Hair restoration surgery affects many aspects of a patient's life. Natural looking results from today's hair transplant surgeries can potentially reverse many psycho social problems associated with hair loss. The positive impact of hair restoration is more visible among patients who suffer from those effects the most. In early stages of hair loss, patients may have more awareness of their condition and they might be more affected than those in the later stages of hair loss.

According to the study, patients who experienced hair loss at an early age, and also had an active social life were, more prone to the negative effects of balding such as anxiety. Therefore, we can assume that hair loss can have a negative impact on a patient's outlook which seems to reverse after receiving a hair restoration procedure.

Although the response rate in our study was not one hundred percent, it supported what hair restoration physicians report from observations and from anecdotal evidence of patients. Efforts are being made to repeat the study in the future on a larger scale. Most importantly, it is clear with the advancements in hair restoration, providing natural results for men and women who suffer from hair loss is crucial.

## FINAL THOUGHTS ON HAIR AND SELF-IMAGE

If you are experiencing hair loss, but it does not negatively impact your life, hair restoration surgery is most likely something you would not choose to do. For most men and women who are suffering from hair loss, hair restoration makes significant improvements in many aspects of their psycho social lives including, but not limited to, their overall happiness, self-esteem, outlook, sex life and career.

Since you are reading this book, it is likely that either you or a loved one might benefit from a professional consultation and evaluation with a hair restoration doctor. Enjoy reading this book as it will answer many of your questions. Most of all, I wish you the best in health and life.

# HAIR LOSS FACTS AND MYTHS

**H**air loss is evident throughout the records of human history. As far back as ancient Egypt, there is anthropological evidence that wigs and hair augmentation of some type was a cultural norm. Though people now live longer thanks to general health improvement, hair loss has yet to be eradicated and still has strong cultural ramifications.

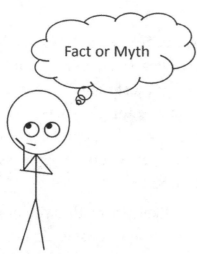

The strong emphasis placed on hair in society sometimes fosters desperateness in people suffering from hair loss. This anxiety causes many people to try pretty much anything and everything that is claimed to be effective. This reason has led to the exploitation of persons with baldness. Unfortunately, the proliferation of myth over fact causes confusion for people who genuinely seek remedy for hair loss. In this chapter, we will present some facts and myths regarding hair loss and hair restoration. If you smile or have a chuckle reading here, it's okay. It's amazing how some myths have been perpetuated.

## HAIR LOSS FACTS

Most doctors will tell you to eat a balanced healthy diet with whole foods from the basic food groups. A healthy dietary intake benefits every aspect of our body. For centuries, healthy hair and skin have been perceived as an indicator of inner health. This is true to a certain extent. A well-balanced diet contributes to feeling and looking well. What a surprise! But let's get to some basic hair loss facts.

1. **Our hair is made of a protein**
   Hair and nails are a variation of skin. They are all forms of a keratinized protein. Hair grows all over the human body. The exceptions are the palms of the hands, soles of the feet and lips.

2. **Only hair root matters**
   A hair consists of a hair shaft (the part we see), a root below the skin and a follicle from which the hair roots grow. It is the damage to the hair follicle that eventually leads to hair loss which is considered a medical condition. This should not be confused with the normal shedding of hair. It is normal to shed hair. Losing 50 to 100 hairs is considered normal. Occasionally, and under special circumstances, this number may go up to 200 hairs per day. There is no need to count those hairs from your brush or comb. Hair loss that demands medical attention is most often perceptibly noticeable.

3. **Color of hair**

The hair color pigment, or melanin, is produced at the hair bulb, which is located at the lower end of the follicle. Therefore, no hair color is truly permanent. Your hair color is programmed genetically over the course of your lifetime. Some environmental factors such as the sun or chlorine can alter hair color but not the color of the hair growing from the follicle.

4. **Hair loss and stress**

The hair shaft falling out or hair shedding could be directly connected to stress. Sometimes that stress is caused by excessive work, family problems or major illness or surgeries. When stress is eliminated, our relieved hair will usually return to its normal growth pattern. However, if you are genetically prone to baldness, stress may hasten something that is going to happen anyway and it might not reversible. It is best to have a medical evaluation when a perceptible level of hair loss occurs.

5. **Hair loss because of hormonal imbalances**

Hair loss can be caused by hormonal problems and correcting the hormone imbalance may stop the hair loss. Hormonal changes are often related to hair loss. The important thing is to learn the root of the hormonal change. Pregnancy and postpartum periods are obvious examples of such conditions that affect hair growth and hair loss. Alteration of both male and female sex hormones may be a cause of hair loss conditions.

Other hormonal problems can be caused by an overactive or underactive thyroid gland.

6. **Hair loss after giving birth**
   Many women experience hair loss in the first few months of giving birth. During pregnancy, high levels of progesterone usually cause the body to keep and grow the hair that was supposed to fall off naturally. It is therefore considered normal that, when the progesterone levels drop to pre-pregnancy levels, the supporting effects of those hormones are gone and hair starts to fall out. The natural hair loss and growth cycle should resume in a few months.

7. **Medications can cause hair loss**
   Hair loss can be caused by certain medicines or treatments. Blood thinners (anticoagulants), gout medicines, chemotherapy (used for cancer treatment), Vitamin A (in large amounts) and some birth control pills and antidepressants have hair loss indicated as a possible side effect. There are many more medications that have hair loss as one of the rare side effects. Don't worry too much if you see hair loss listed in the problems that may happen after taking any medications. Just discuss it with your doctor to see how relevant it is to your current condition. Hair loss should usually stop when you stop taking the medicines. Your doctor may suggest a change of medicines or treatment that won't cause you the hair loss.

8. **Fungus and hair loss**

Hair loss can be caused by fungal infections of the scalp. These conditions can be treated with anti-fungal medicines. A physician should be seen as soon as possible.

9. **My immune system causing my hair loss**

Hair loss can be caused by an autoimmune disease known as alopecia areata (AA). AA is caused by an overreaction of one's own immune system. It initially appears as small, round and coin shaped bald patches on the scalp which can get bigger in some cases. The hair often grows back natu-rally within six months to a year in most cases but those patients might experience that kind of alopecia again.

10. **Hair loss can be a result of poor nutrition.**

Anorexic and bulimic people experience hair loss because their body does not get the necessary nutrients needed for many bodily functions. Hair loss that leads to typical patterned baldness is most often not from nutrition but from a significant stressor along with genetics. This is discussed in detail in upcoming chapters.

11. **Causes of typical men hair loss**

A very frequent kind of hair loss (alopecia) is commonly called male pattern baldness or, in medical terms, androgenic alopecia. This is caused by genetic factors but can be accelerated by a com-bination of many other factors including stress, medications and hormonal changes.

## 12. Good diet cannot stop hair loss

Eating a healthy balanced diet is good for your health and general well-being. This is true in the sense that a good dietary intake provides the body with the nutrients it needs to function properly. However, your patterned hair loss is not associated with your nutrition. There is no diet that is known to stop patterned hair loss. Balding will eventually occur despite having a balanced diet.

## 13. Shampoo and hair loss

Some doctors advise their patients to use baby shampoo and not to wash their hair more than once a day. The thought here is to use gentle hair care products. Some hair care cosmetics are harsh and damage your hair despite their claims to be helping your hair loss. However, this is not the main cause of patterned hair loss. Your genetics most often are.

## 14. Pulling hair can cause permanent hair loss

Puling hair on a regular basis, as in people who do tight braids or the ones using tight turbines, can cause a special form of hair loss called traction alopecia. You should avoid anything that pulls your hair continuously for prolonged periods of time.

## 15. Hair loss is a disease

Hair loss is a common disease but, because it is so common in men, we generally do not take it seriously. If you experience unexplained hair loss or you have a genetic factor that might cause you to lose your hair, seeing a medical doctor is the best thing to do to determine the cause of your hair loss.

It is advisable to consult a doctor before starting any over the counter medications that might be available without prescription.

16. **Styling can damage hair**

    Styling hair with rollers and irons, vigorously brushing, pulling or tight braiding, as mentioned before, can cause damage to hair shafts or even hair follicles. However, damaging the hair shaft should not be mistaken with typical male or female hair loss.

17. **You can avoid chemical damage to your hair**

    You should always test chemical hair processes before applying them to your hair. When using products such as relaxers, permanents or hair color, you should first try them on a small section on the back of both skin and hair to check for allergies and hair loss or damage. After a successful test, wait a few days and then have the process on your entire hair and scalp. It is always better to have them done by a trained and licensed professional.

18. **Steroids can cause hair loss**

    Some medications are known to have the side effect of hair loss. Anabolic steroids are well-known for this. Though they might not cause hair loss for someone who isn't genetically predisposed to hair loss, this group of steroids can exacerbate balding tendencies in someone who is genetically susceptible to male pattern baldness.

**19. Genes are the main cause of hair loss**
It is important to note that hereditary hair loss is responsible for almost all patterned hair losses and it is not affected by nutrition to any perceptible level. If hair loss is due to nutritional/dietary deficiency then improving nutrition will most likely cause the hair loss to abate.

**20. Hair loss may be related to depression**
Many people normally experience depression when they start losing hair. Scientific research shows us that people with hair loss have higher rates of depression. Many people with situational baldness or female/male pattern baldness suffer in private. If this is you, then you should not despair because the condition can be improved by hair restoration. For more on this you can review our article, "Psychology of Hair Transplant."[4]

**21. Mineral deficiency can cause hair loss**
Acute deficiency of some minerals may cause hair loss or thinning, dermatitis and slow hair growth. Zinc is one of the minerals that may cause hair loss in its severe form. Both poor appetite and poor digestion are also experienced by adults with a zinc deficiency. Iron deficiency can also cause hair loss in a diffuse form. Iron deficiency can also accelerate the rate of hair loss if you're predisposed to other types of hair loss such as patterned alopecia.

### 22. Stress can cause hair loss

Stress is directly related to hair loss and is one of the primary causes of thinning hair. Hair loss induced by stress can be caused by physical or emotional stress. After severe stressors, such as surgery, trauma or illness, hair loss can occur. This type of hair loss is referred to as Telogen Effluvium or TE. Telogen Effluvium is when a large number of hair follicles decide to go to the resting phase at the same time. TE often takes as long as four to six months to reverse itself.

### 23. Hair loss can cause social anxiety

As mentioned above, stress could be related to hair loss and may accelerate it. Some studies show that hair loss can cause anxiety especially in young adults who suffer from patterned hair loss. The way we look is very important in the social life of young adults and losing hair in those socially active years could be devastating. Our studies show that hair restorations have been able to improve anxiety in young adults.

### 24. Hair loss can affect sex

Our study, that is published in hair transplant forum international, reveals that most people who had a hair restoration reported a significant improvement in their overall sex life.

---

4. Psychology of hair transplant, Parsa Mohebi, MD and William Rassman, MD, Hair Transplant Forum International, the Journal of International Society of Hair Restoration Surgery, cover article, Volume 18, Number 2, March/April 2008

# HAIR LOSS MYTHS

Hair loss is a very common occurrence throughout the world. It spares no social strata, culture or ethnicity. Fortunately, the latest technologies in hair restoration provide solutions that help hair loss sufferers to regain confidence in their self-image. The root causes of hair loss are varied with the most common being male patterned hair loss and female patterned hair loss.

Let's take a moment and clear up some of the common myths or misconceptions that we hear every day in our hair restoration centers. This is an interactive chapter. You might have some fun noting in pencil which ones you have heard before and which ones you think are true or false! By the time you finish reading, you will definitely know what the myths are.

*May we have a drum roll please, presenting ...*

## *The Greatest Hair Loss Myths*

1. **Too much shampooing contributes to hair loss**
   A clean healthy scalp is good. It is okay to have a little 'OCD' about real clean hair. This will not make your hair fall out. Shampooing can be based on the type of work environment you are in as well as the secretions of oils by your body.

2. **Hats and wigs cause hair loss**
   This is based on the flawed reasoning that poor oxygenation is at the root cause of hair loss. This is simply not true. Hair follicles need oxygen but they get it from blood circulation and not from skin surface.

3. **Shaving your infant's head will make hair grow thicker**

You really must wonder how this one came about. In many cultures, it is traditional to shave the baby's head during a ceremonial ritual. Many babies are born with little and very uneven hair. When you shave, you lose the tapering end of hair and you can see the tip of new hair is coarser. Hair cutting or shaving at any age does not promote hair growth.

4. **Coloring and other hair cosmetic treatments cause permanent hair loss**

This is simply not true. Hair coloring only affects the hair shafts that are dead parts of hair and hair follicles are not affected in any way by coloring or chemically processing hair. Chemical treatments, combined with long term tight hairstyles such as braiding, or plaiting can lead to traction alopecia. However, it does not cause pattern baldness.

5. **Women are expected to develop thicker hair**

Women in general seem to grow hair longer than men. However, color and thickness of hair is hereditary and varies from person to person.

6. **We lose hair because of lack of blood circulation**

Hair follicles obtain their oxygen and nutrients from blood circulation but typical patterned hair loss among men and women has nothing to do with circulatory problems. If the balding area of scalp had less blood supply, a hair transplant could not bring hair back to the bald area. If it did, transplanted hair would be prone to baldness too.

We know that transplanted hair follows the pattern of hair growth of the donor area and is not affected by the genetic pattern of baldness.

7. **Standing on one's head will stimulate hair growth**

As mentioned above, patterned baldness is not secondary to circulation problems. If this were true, the vast amount of middle age men with hair loss would lose their bellies, buff up their torsos and walk to work on their arms. If you start seeing this in your locale then there has been a great scientific revelation. However, this is highly unlikely.

8. **Dandruff causes permanent hair loss**

Excessively dry scalp can lead to a buildup of epithelial cells on the scalp that flake off but have nothing to do with hair loss. Nevertheless, severe dandruff may require the evaluation of a dermatologist. The cause of hair loss is not topical or epidermal.

9. **There are cosmetic products that will grow hair faster**

Well, everyone losing hair has fallen for this one most likely and a lot of folks have made a lot of money and still do. This is simply a fallacy. If it was true, the millions and millions of hair loss suffers would not be bald! There are some medically approved solutions such as minoxidil that can slow down the process of balding. Some cosmetics may have these as their active ingredients. If you want to utilize these medications, it is better to use them pure and not as an addition to a shampoo or other cosmetic product.

10. **Permanent hair loss is the result of stress**
Hair loss can be accelerated by stress. However, in most cases when the stress is relieved, hair returns to its normal growth cycle in six to twelve months.

11. **Typical male hair loss starts after twenties**
Unfortunately, the hormonal changes at puberty can affect hair loss in some adolescent males and, in rare circumstances, females. It may not be completely apparent but microscopic evaluation, or a miniaturization study, can reveal the early signs of patterned hair loss even in mid to late teens.

12. **Hair loss affects intellectuals more**
Remember all those men walking to work on their arms earlier? They took a special medication called 'Low IQ"! Nope, this is a myth. You can have a prolific head of hair and not the intellect to match…imagine that!

13. **Androgenic Alopecia can be cured**
Hair restoration and some medications are the only proven methods of alleviating the effects of androgenic alopecia. As of now, there is not a cure for male patterned baldness.

14. **Wearing a tight baseball cap too often will make you bald**
This is the poor circulation concept in hat form. Total Myth! However, there is a condition called turbine alopecia that is seen mostly in Indians who wear very tight turbines for most of their lives. That is a type of traction alopecia that will be discussed later. I have never seen it happening with baseball caps!

15. **Brushing helps you grow hair**

The idea of brushing the hair 100 times a day to stimulate the scalp circulation is a fantasy. In fact, if you brush your hair too much, you may end up traumatizing your hair shafts. This myth stems from the thought that hair loss was due to poor circulation and that brushing, or massaging, would improve blood flow and nutrition to the follicles. The truth is, bald or not, there's no major difference in scalp circulation.

16. **Styling causes hair loss**

There is some truth and some fiction when it comes to hairstyling and hair loss. It is true that certain hairstyles, such as cornrows or tight ponytails for long periods, can cause hair loss. These styles put undue tension on the hair. As for hair sprays, perm solutions, or coloring resulting in hair loss, there's no truth to that idea. These applications may cause some damage to the hair strands. But the important areas of hair follicles, located under the skin, stay safe.

17. **More frequent haircuts will make your hair grow faster**

That is wishful thinking. Everyone's hair growth and length depend on their own unique hair cycle which is primarily heredity. The longer your hair growth phase, the longer your hair growth. Your hair follicles have no way of knowing how long your hair shaft is.

18. **Blow drying your hair will cause your hair to thin out**

There is no evidence that hair dryers cause thinning hair Over drying can lead to damage that renders your hair brittle and more breakable. Hold the hair dryer at a distance from your scalp well enough to dry it but not to scorch it.

19. **Vitamins will make your hair grow**
    If you are losing hair because of a lack of vitamins or minerals in your diet, why wouldn't the back and sides of your head be affected? Vitamin deficiency usually results in an even distribution of hair loss all over the head, i.e. thinning of the hair. It does not hurt to take vitamins on a regular basis for your overall health especially in certain conditions that are recommended by doctors. Your follicle width and amount are based on heredity. So, claims of hair growing miracle drugs or natural hair loss treatments are untrue to that extent. Improved nutrition helps the whole body within its genetic predisposition.

20. **Steroids can help your hair grow better**
    Anabolic steroids can cause hair loss. Research has proven that anabolic steroids raise the levels of baldness-inducing male hormones. For those who are genetically prone to hair loss, this can speed up the loss in as little as three to six months. While this loss may be reversed, it can be permanent in some cases.

21. **Sexual activity increases hair growth**
    Wishful thinking folks... there is no truth to the idea that the more sex you have, the less hair you will lose! Or that the chemicals released during sex can affect hair loss. The opposite is not true either. Science has yet to uncover any proof to these

fantasies. But that doesn't mean you shouldn't keep conducting your own clinical trials (wink.)

22. **My father has a great head of hair so I have no worries**

Many men believe that if their father has a full head of hair, they will keep a good head of hair. Nonetheless, hair loss or hair growth is set by a genetic combination determined by both sides of your family. Of course, if your family tree is filled with balding scalps, you do have a better chance of losing hair.

23. **Baldness is passed down from your mother's side**

Hereditary hair loss, or androgenic alopecia, is considered the main cause of hair loss in women and in men. It accounts for 95% of male hair loss. Long considered a trait inherited from our mother's side, genetic hair loss actually results from a combination of the genes from our mother's and our father's sides. Although you cannot entirely predict the future of your hairline based on your mother's or your father's scalp, you can get a good indicator from comparing the collective hairlines of your parents, grandparents, aunts and uncles.

24. **Tightness of scalp can be the cause of hair loss**

This is not true. During a pre-op evaluation, we examine scalp laxity with a device called the Laxometer. We have seen a range of very loose to very tight scalps among balding people and there has not been a significant relationship between scalp tightness and hair loss. Therefore, you can probably guess that scalp massage cannot help that recessing hair line of yours either but it can lead to some enjoyable life moments!

**25. Stress is the main cause of hair loss in men**

While none of these symptoms are known to create permanent hair loss, they can all create significant temporary hair loss in men and women. When it comes to vitamin or nutritional deficiency and intense stress, the resulting temporary hair loss is called Telogen Effluvium. This hair loss happens when the body experiences a shock, either from psychological stress, sudden excessive weight loss, metabolic changes, vitamin deficiencies or a virus. When one of these situations occurs, the hair is forced into the resting stage of the hair growth cycle prematurely which results in sudden drastic hair loss. However, it is not the typical hair loss men experience as male patterned baldness.

**26. Using a night cap can prevent hair loss**

Some people have maintained that keeping the scalp covered during night or day can increase blood flow of the scalp and boost hair growth. Because alopecia is primarily caused by the presence of DHT and genetic pre-disposition, rather than blood flow, using night hats won't have any effect on your hair.

**27. Regular shaving makes your hair regenerate faster**

Getting frequent haircuts or shaving your head might be considered a good way to keep existing hair healthy by removing damaged, split ends. However, haircuts have no effect on your hair's growth rate or thickness overall. It is simply the duration of a person's unique hair growth phase.

## 28. Smoking causes hair loss

Although this myth has been discounted in the past as being an invalid assumption, a thirty-year study by the research group, the British Medical Journal (BMJ)5 have found sufficient evidence to claim there might be a link between smoking and hair loss. It's still uncertain whether the connection is because of tobacco toxins or the fact that smoking accelerates aging and other health problems. So, although this is not quite a myth, we wanted to get your attention about another hazard of smoking!

## 29. Hair loss cannot be treated

In the past, there were no effective treatments in sight for hair loss and hair thinning patients. The only solution was to cover up hair loss with hats and artificial hairpieces. Fortunately, there are many effective hair loss medications and treatments in today's market that can either prevent future hair loss or replenish balding hairlines. The most popular hair loss medications include Rogaine® (minoxidil) and Propecia® (finasteride). Rogaine acts as a hair growth stimulator while Propecia prevents hair loss by inhibiting DHT production and activity. There is more on hair loss medications in that section of this book. Those medications are mostly to prevent or slow down hair loss but hair transplantation can restore a balding head by relocating hair from areas with permanent hair growth to balding portions permanently. Today this is absolutely a myth.

---

5. BMJ 1996; 313 doi: 10.1136/bmj.313.7072.1616 (Published 21 December 1996)

## 30. I have to wait till I am completely bald before I can have a hair transplant

In the past, hair transplant surgeons did not perform a hair transplant before patients were in their mid-twenties. Some surgeons refused to perform hair restoration before a person lost all of his or her hair. Today we know that hair restoration can be done at any age as long as we can determine the final pattern of hair loss with microscopic evaluation and through family history of balding. Hair transplant surgeons do not have to wait for you to go completely bald before performing a hair transplant. In fact we would like to perform a hair transplant before anyone knows you are balding. Medical treatments could be added to hair restoration to preserve your native hair in balding areas. The combination of surgery and medical treatments of hair loss can change what was known to be your hair destiny.

Well, there you have it! Some serious hair restoration facts and myths! These are some of the common myths heard by hair loss specialists on a daily basis. It is recommended that you first have your hair loss diagnosed by a competent hair loss expert. Hair transplant surgeons are medical doctors who see hair loss patients regularly. Once you have received a thorough evaluation and consultation, you will have a better understanding of exactly which treatment options are available and what may be best for you.

# NORMAL HAIR GROWTH CYCLE

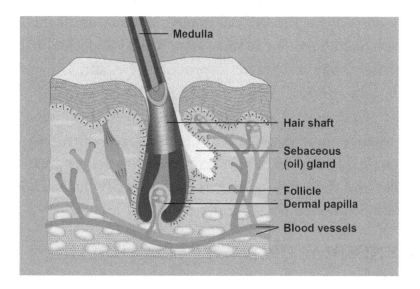

**The basic factors a person should know to better understand hair loss are:**

- Understanding hair structure
- Understanding the hair growth cycle

## HAIR STRUCTURE

Hair is composed of durable resistant structural protein called keratin. Keratin is the same kind of protein that makes up the nails and the epidermis (outer layer of skin.)

There are three layers of each hair strand. These layers are:
- The Medulla is the core innermost layer
- The Cortex provides color, strength, and texture
- The Cuticle is the thin and colorless outermost layer of hair

## STRUCTURE OF THE HAIR ROOT

The hair root lies beneath the skin's surface and is contained in a hair follicle. The dermal papilla is made up of the base of the hair follicle. The bloodstream feeds the dermal papilla which carries nourishment to produce new hair. The importance of the dermal papilla is magnified as the receptors for male hormones and androgens are within it. It is androgens that regulate hair growth. It is the androgen dihydrotestosterone (DHT) that causes the hair follicle to get progressively smaller and the hairs to become finer in individuals who are genetically predisposed to this type of hair loss.

## THE NORMAL GROWTH CYCLE OF HAIR

There are three phases of the hair growth cycle:

| Normal Hair Growth Cycle | | |
|---|---|---|
| Phase | Function | Duration |
| Anagen | Growth | 2 - 8 years |
| Catagen | Degradation | 2 - 4 weeks |
| Telogen | Resting | 2 - 4 months |

*On average 50-100 telogen hairs (resting phase) are shed every day. This is normal everyday hair loss found in our comb or the shower. These hairs regrow in the anagen phase. About ten percent of the follicles are in the resting phase (telogen) in a given period of time. Medically this is referred to as shedding; it is just normal hair loss.*

There are various factors that affect the normal hair growth cycle and cause temporary or permanent hair loss (alopecia) including medication, radiation, chemotherapy, exposure to chemicals, hormonal and nutritional factors, thyroid disease, generalized or local skin disease and stress.

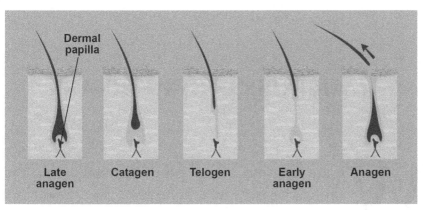

Androgens are the most important factor in hair growth. These hormones are testosterone and dihydrotestosterone (DHT). It is the presence of androgens that fosters the beard and the growth of auxiliary hair underarms and pubic hair. Scalp hair is not androgen dependent but androgens are the underlying cause that initiates the genetic predisposition of male and female pattern hair loss otherwise referred to as Male Pattern Baldness (MPB) and Female Pattern Baldness (FPB). Medical science advances in recent years have elevated medical hair restoration and hair transplant surgery as a preferable option for men and women. Hair restoration is a highly successful method for treating MPB and FPB.

# HAIR LOSS IS HEREDITARY

We are the sum of our genes in many ways. Even though we may favor one parent over the other, as we become more acquainted with different family members on both sides, we start to find common traits with various members from our families. Though certainly one parental side may be more dominant over the other, our hair and the loss thereof, to a significant point, is also hereditary.

Perhaps you know someone in their teens or early twenties who has started to experience thinning hair. The odds are the culprit is hidden in that complex of genetic code we call our 'family tree.' Nearly ninety five percent of men and seventy percent of women with thinning hair can attribute it to a hereditary condition called Androgenic Alopecia (male or female patterned baldness). In layman terms, it is referred to as male patterned baldness (MPB) in men and female pattern baldness (FPB) in women.

Hair loss is an equal opportunity culprit. Androgenic Alopecia affects all ethnicities and can be inherited from either the paternal or maternal side of the family. There are numerous genetic factors that determine baldness. It may or may not skip generations.

***Hereditary hair loss is characterized by:***
- a progressive miniaturization of hair follicles
- a shortening of the hair's growth cycle

As the growth phase shortens, the hair becomes thinner and shorter until, eventually, there is no growth at all.

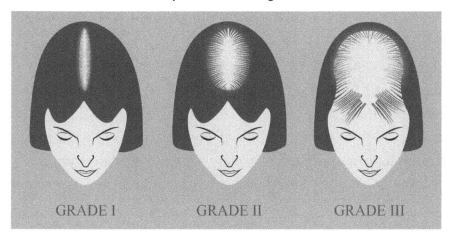

*Female Patterned Baldness*

The most common type of hair loss in men and women, or pattern baldness, is a condition that is a result of some combination of genetics, hormonal changes and the aging process. Among all, genetics is the most important factor contributing to one's hair loss. Hereditary pattern is also known as patterned baldness. Patterned baldness is most often referred to as male patterned baldness (MPB) in men and female pattern baldness (FPB) in typical female hair loss. The incidence of MPB6 far exceeds that of FPB.7

Medical science, developments and advancements in hair restoration have made male pattern and female pattern Androgenic Alopecia a treatable condition with very successful results. Improved self-image and esteem that men and women gain through successful hair restoration is beneficially life changing.

MPB and FPB are so common that today's medical professionals have been paying more attention which has been leading to the boom in advancements in hair transplantation. These surgical and medical hair loss treatments have high rates of success.

Hereditary hair loss is gradual but, the sooner treatment is started, the better the chances of results that will please the patient throughout the course of their life. Checking your family tree to see if you have a possible genetic predisposition to hair loss might help you recognize the symptoms early enough to slow the progression with today's FDA approved medications.

The advances in research have helped medical professionals to better understand the cause of this most common type of hair loss and balding genes. Under the influence of a form of the male hormone, the normal cycle of hair growth changes in hair follicles, that are genetically prone to baldness, results in shorter, thinner or "miniaturized" hair. Later in this book, we will learn more about this common hereditary challenge and hair miniaturization process.

# MEN'S HAIR LOSS IS MULTICULTURAL

Hair loss affects up to 60% of the male population in every ethnicity. This common worldwide phenomenon is also referred to as male patterned baldness (MPB.) The past decade has brought forth advancements in medical science and medical technology making resolving MPB a viable option for many men through hair restoration.

Modern hair restoration through hair transplantation provides a natural, proven and permanent solution for men. Hair transplants are now one of the most common cosmetic procedures chosen by men today.

# CAUSES OF BALDNESS IN MEN

### *The Most Common Cause of Baldness in Men*
Hormonal and genetic factors both play a role but the exact root mechanism for baldness in men is still being researched by medical science. This will affect more men by each decade of their life. Male Pattern Baldness affects 20% of men in their twenties, 30% of men in their thirties, 40% of men in their forties and so forth. MPB Hair loss can begin even in the later stages of puberty. The Hamilton-Norwood scale is used for the classification of male pattern baldness and is based on the progress and severity of hair loss. Currently, several treatment options are available. Besides hair transplantation, there are two medications that have been FDA-approved for use in the United States. Patients who benefit the most from the effects of medications on slowing the balding process are still in the initial stages of baldness.

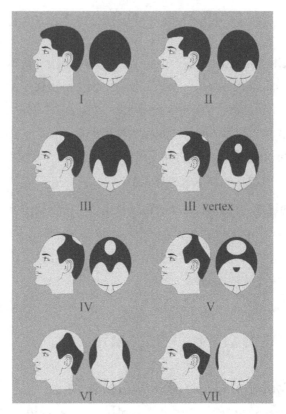

*Hair loss classifications for men with MPB*

Research has proven that the prime culprit in MPB is dihydrotestosterone (DHT) which is a powerful sex hormone known to adversely affect hair follicles in the crown, top and temples of the scalp. DHT is clinically verified as the trigger for male pattern baldness. In addition, researchers noted that men with MPB also have elevated levels of the enzyme 5 alpha-reductase.

The act of genes, hormones and time makes the susceptible hair follicles in those regions of the scalp produce shorter and finer hair over time. When no medical intervention takes place, these follicles will eventually cease to produce hair shafts at all. This process is called miniaturization. The progress of this miniaturization causes the disappearance of certain hair shafts and shrinkage of the others. In this process, the scalp hair becomes very fine and short and is also known as miniaturized hair.

## TREATMENT OF MALE PATTERN BALDNESS (MPB)

The centuries old medical treatment for baldness in men is a longstanding historical challenge. Finally, for the first time in history, FDA approved medications are having measurable effects on pattern hair loss in men. These results vary from person to person but are successful enough to garner FDA approval.

### *SOME OF THE DRUGS INCLUDE:*

### *Minoxidil (Rogaine)*
It is one of two Food and Drug Administration (FDA) approved medications and it comes in a topical form. Minoxidil is available in 2% and 5% solutions. It needs to be applied to the balding areas of the scalp and its effectiveness is usually not noticeable for several months after initiation of treatment. Positive results of the medication are not permanent, and, in most cases, the patient will still experience hair loss after the medication has been discontinued. Hair transplant surgeons may recommend the use of minoxidil along with hair transplantation as a compliment for successful hair restoration.

### Finasteride (Propecia)

This is the only available oral medication for male pattern baldness. It is available for hair loss treatment in one milligram pills and one pill should be taken every day. In the absence of a hair transplant, withdrawal from finasteride usually leads to reversal of hair loss within 12 months.

### Hair Transplant

Hair transplant is the natural, proven and permanent treatment for baldness in men. Formerly, surgical treatments such as plug grafts, scalp flaps and scalp reductions were used with less than desirable results for patients. The advancement and discovery of Follicular Unit Transplant (FUT) revolutionized hair restoration treatment of hair loss for both men and women.

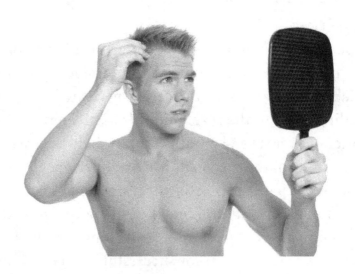

# OTHER CAUSES OF HAIR LOSS IN MEN

## *Alopecia Areata*
Alopecia areata is an autoimmune disease that affects hair follicles anywhere in the body and appears as round patches without hair. Alopecia areata affects both men and women and can be seen almost anywhere on the skin.

## *Anagen Effluvium*
This refers to sudden hair loss due to the effect of chemicals or radiations such as hair loss following chemotherapy, radiation therapy or toxins. This condition is different from Telogen effluvium where hair enters the resting phase. In this condition, hair loss begins 1-3 weeks following exposure to the inducing factor. Some types of anagen effluvium such as hair loss after chemotherapy could be temporary and hair growth is back to normal once treatment is finished. The texture of hair could be somehow different after regrowth in some cases.

## *Trichotillomania*
Trichotillomania is a hair loss condition in which patients continuously pull hair causing hair loss in some areas. This condition is usually an outgrowth of an underlying emotional and psychological disorder such as anxiety. Trichotillomania most commonly occurs among children and adolescents. Women are affected twice as much as men. People affected by it may pull hair from any part of the body including the eyebrows, beard and body hair.

## *Traction Alopecia*
Traction Alopecia is caused by continuous pulling on the hair when styling it. This pulling causes local hair loss in the affected area. The factors such as various hairstyles, ponytails

and tight braiding are often a root cause. The process of hair loss is gradual but, if the cause continues, the hair loss can become permanent. Permanent types of traction alopecia can be successfully treated with hair transplantation.

### Telogen Effluvium

Hair loss can happen suddenly like in the case of Telogen Effluvium. It is usually stress related hair loss which appears as general thinning throughout the scalp. Telogen Effluvium can occur after any severe and sudden stress. In Telogen Effluvium, a large number of hair follicles enter the resting (telogen) phase at once causing general hair loss or thinning over large areas of the scalp. In most cases, the hair loss recovers spontaneously and completely. Telogen Effluvium can be seen in patients who are prone to male or female patterned baldness and stress can cause accelerated hair loss that may be not reversible due to underlying conditions. The most common form of Telogen Effluvium is seen after childbirth or pregnancy termination in women.

### Shock Loss after Surgery

The stress and physical changes following major surgeries or procedures of head and scalp area can cause sudden hair loss in the involved areas. This is known as shock loss. Hair transplant used to be one of the major causes of shock loss but using medication such as finasteride (Propecia) has reduced the rate of hair loss after hair transplant surgeries significantly.

### Medication Induced Hair Loss

Many medications have hair loss as one of their side effects but here is a list of the most important ones:

- Chemotherapy medications
- Allopurinol
- Coumarin
- Clofibrate
- Gemfibrozil
- Heparin

## *Scarring Alopecia*

Scarring alopecia can be caused by gross scars such as surgical incisions or traumatic injuries. It could happen at the cellular level by inflammatory reactions such as skin infections destroying hair follicles. "Alopecia" is a condition in which patients lose hair in part or all of the head or body due to destruction of hair follicles at the cellular level. Cicatricial alopecia generally happens following a skin infection or inflammatory process. Scarring alopecia is a result of surgical incisions or trauma and can be easily treated with hair transplantation or sometimes with a simple excision of the scar.

## *Infections and Hair Loss*

Infection used to be one of the most common causes of hair loss in children in the past but is seen very rarely now thanks to the effective antibiotic and antifungal treatments that can cure scalp infectious diseases.

# WOMEN'S HAIR LOSS

Given the significance of hair and its relation to a woman's beauty in our society, hair loss in women can be even more devastating as compared to men. However, hair loss in women is a more complex medical issue. There are various causes for the interruption of the normal hair growth in women.

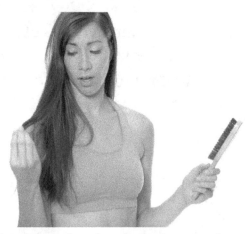

The average rate of hair growth is about one centimeter per month. The normal hair growth cycle consists of three phases; anagen (growth), catagen (transitional) and telogen (resting) phase. This lifecycle of scalp hair can take approximately 2 to 6 years to be completed for a single follicle. After the falling of hair, a new hair grows in its place. In a normal person, 85 percent of hair is growing at any given time and the other 15 percent is resting.

The growth cycle of normal hair can change in women with hormonal changes. Most women grow their hair better during pregnancy and lose some hair after delivery of a baby. This condition is called Telogen Effluvium, which is one of the most common causes of hair loss in young women. This condition is always reversible unless the person has other underlying causes for her hair loss.

## MINIATURIZATION IN WOMEN

Baldness is a condition in which new hair does not grow when old hair falls or the new hair is miniaturized. Miniaturization is a state where the new hair is finer and or thinner. Miniaturization could be a precursor of hair loss and could be diagnosed with microscopic evaluation of hair and scalp. Why women lose the thickness of their hair shaft, and eventually lose their hair in female pattern baldness (FPB), is not entirely understood. Presently, it is understood that female hair loss in the form of male or female patterned baldness are associated with genetics, hormonal changes and aging. Hormonal changes are commonly seen in pregnancy, the menopausal period and some endocrine imbalances.

## PATTERNS OF FEMALE HAIR LOSS

Most women lose their hair in a specific pattern that could be classified into Male Patterned Baldness (MPB) or Female Patterned Baldness (FPB). Both of these conditions are often caused by hormones, aging, and other genetic factors.

Female patterned baldness generally differs from male pattern baldness. In female pattern baldness, the hair thins out more diffusely. It can also follow a central thinning that may expand to involve the entire scalp. Most women may maintain their hairline to some degree. Male Patterned Baldness usually presents itself with a recession from front and frontal corners and temple areas. It also may present itself with isolated crown balding as it could be seen in some men. Female pattern baldness can occasionally appear similar to male pattern baldness but it rarely progresses to full or even near total baldness, as it does in men.

## PATTERNS IN WOMEN'S HAIR LOSS

*Typical patterns of hair loss in women are:*

1. Diffuse thinning with thinning in donor hair on the back and sides (FPB).

2. These groups of patients are generally not good candidates for a hair transplant procedure due to instability of their donor area. Medical treatment should be considered as the first line of treatment.

3. Less diffuse hair thinning with protected donor hair. More noticeable thinning is seen in some areas such as front, corners and crown areas (MPB).

4. Patients in this group have the best results from hair transplant since they have intact donor hair. Medical evaluation should be performed to check the hormonal levels and, in particular, testosterone levels.

5. Diffuse thinning with more noticeable thinning towards the front of the scalp. Involvement, and sometimes breaching, of the frontal hairline can be noticed. This group can also be treated like MPB group with hair

transplant if the donor hair is intact.

6. Diffused Unpatterned Alopecia (DUPA) in which hair becomes thin diffusely without following any specific pattern. This pattern that can be seen in both men and women generally does not leave the patient with any intact hair on donor areas. These patients are generally not good candidates for hair transplant.

# OVERALL MANAGEMENT OF WOMEN'S HAIR LOSS

After treating women with hair loss for many years, we have established a protocol for management of women with hair loss. This approach gives a simple outline for diagnosis and treatment of many hair loss conditions in women.

## Step 1: History

An accurate and complete history of hair loss is the foremost factor in treatment and management of women's hair loss. This should include:

- family history of hair loss especially in members of the same gender
- other previous and present medical problems
- medications that are used by the patient

When a strong family history for female hair loss is not present, it is less likely that the patient will be suffering from FPB. Various types of medications are known for having hair loss as one of their side effects. This is why it is important that the patient's history of medications be carefully evaluated. However, many women do not lose hair solely after the use of medications.

### *Step 2: Macro and Micro-evaluation*

Thorough scalp examination by a hair transplant surgeon should be done carefully to examine the scalp and determine the presence of abnormal pattern of hair loss. A woman presenting classic male pattern hair loss (MPB) such as a receding hairline, or significant thinning in front with preserved hair on sides and back, should be evaluated for elevated testosterone levels.

Microscopic evaluation of the scalp and hair (miniaturization study) is an important part of every hair loss evaluation in both men and women. Microscopic evaluation guides a hair restoration specialist in monitoring the patient's response to medical treatment.

This includes using magnification to look for the presence of very fine hair shafts in the areas of concern.

A small number of fine hairs are normally observed in people due to the natural growth cycle of hair follicles. Miniaturization (fineness) of more than twenty percent of hair shafts cannot be explained by the growth cycle of hair and other causes should be considered. The next step is the mapping of scalp hair miniaturization for all patients during their physical evaluation. This is comparing the numbers of miniaturization after months of treating patients with medication showing the effectiveness of medical treatment. Miniaturization and mapping of hair miniaturization is a verifiable guideline to evaluate the success of hair loss treatments.

In patients who are not qualified for medical therapy, miniaturization could be used to predict the future of their hair loss. This helps a hair transplant surgeon to realize which areas to restore after foreseeing the rate of loss in different areas.

### Step 3: Lab Work

Conducting lab work might be necessary for many women with hair loss. Since hormonal imbalances can be the reason of hair loss and thinning in many women, some hormonal evaluations should be included in hair loss evaluations in women too. The primary hormonal levels to check are total and free testosterone, DHEA sulfate, Prolactin, T3, T4 and TSH. There might be a need to check other specific tests, such as ANA, if there is any evidence of autoimmune disorders that may be associated with hair loss.

In more atypical patterns of hair loss, or in hair loss conditions without a specific family history, the doctor may need to obtain a scalp biopsy to rule out other and rarer skin conditions that may lead to a woman's hair loss. Those conditions include autoimmune conditions of the scalp that cause hair loss such as Alopecia Areata (AA) or Alopecia Cicatricial among others. Confirming the diagnosis of those conditions helps a physician know what type of treatment should or should not be used.

### Step 4: Diagnosis

Treatment of female hair loss is directly related to diagnosis of their hair loss condition. If we diagnose any medical condition that causes hair loss in women, we can treat that condition. In many instances, discovering the cause of hair loss can alleviate the condition through resolving the underlying cause. In cases where we cannot find any other medical condition causing hair loss, which is majority of the cases, we treat female hair loss based on our findings in our macro and microscopic evaluation.

### *Step 5: Treatment*

Diffuse hair loss is the most common type of hair loss in women where the patients have significant thinning or miniaturization of hair throughout scalp. If these women still have high levels of miniaturization (fineness of scalp hair), they generally are good candidates for medical treatment with minoxidil (Rogaine) or similar medications. Baldness could be completed. That means the patient has lost a vast majority of her hair despite having less than 20% miniaturization in the scalp hair. Patients with completed hair loss do not respond to the medical treatment.

Local hair loss, or asymmetrical hair loss with loss of one area (usually the front), and preserving the donor hair on the permanent zone makes women great candidates for hair transplantation. Women's hair transplant surgery can be very successful provided the patients are selected properly by following the other three steps described above.

As with all hair restoration patients, it is important to set the expectations appropriately for women with hair loss. It is crucial to make sure the patient has a good understanding of the final outcome. The level of satisfaction in women with female patterned hair loss may be quite different than with men with male patterned baldness. The importance of providing information with realistic expectations cannot be overemphasized. Women should be informed that, in some cases, more than one hair transplant procedure may be necessary to achieve the best cosmetic result.

It is important to evaluate women's hair loss thoroughly and provide the right diagnosis. Quite often in women's hair loss, medical treatments are used to maintain their hair rather than treating their hair loss.

Producing the original density or something close to it might be more challenging in women with extensive hair loss. Hair restoration surgery for the qualified female candidate can be a positive and uplifting life changing experience.

The combination of medical treatment, hair transplantation and cosmetic changes can help create the appearance of maximum fullness in many women who suffer from female hair loss.

## OTHER CAUSES OF HAIR LOSS IN WOMEN

There are factors other than genetic and hormonal causes of hair loss in women. Female hair loss can also be accelerated by other factors such as:

- Telogen Effluvium – a temporary shedding of hair at a more than usual rate. This is a common cause of hair loss for men and women. This type of accelerated hair loss is not uncommon after the delivery of a baby or any other stressful event.
- Instrumental breaking of hair (usually from aggressive hairstyling treatments)
- Alopecia areata - patchy areas of total hair loss usually facilitated by an immune disorder causing local hair loss.
- Scarring alopecia - patchy hair loss due to infection, inflammation or injury this is often followed by scarring.
- Trichotillomania – compulsive pulling of hair due to anxiety or other psychological issues. Anxiety and signs of compulsive disorder are seen in these patients.
- Hair loss as a side effect of some medications.
- Other skin disorders such as lupus.

# MEDICAL TREATMENT OF WOMEN'S HAIR LOSS

Prior to treating the hair loss, all common treatable causes have to be excluded through lab testing. Rogaine (topical minoxidil 2%) is often prescribed as the first step in medical treatment of these patients. Rogaine is the only FDA-approved medication that is currently available for the medical treatment of female hair loss. Rogaine generally works better in patients who still have active hair loss. The presence of this condition can be confirmed by a microscopic evaluation of scalp. This is a very important reason why patients should only start Rogaine after being evaluated by a hair loss specialist. Nonetheless, not every woman with hair loss responds to Rogaine.

Propecia, the other FDA-approved hair loss treatment for males, has not been proven to demonstrate positive results in women. The exception to this rule is when women lose hair due to elevated levels of testosterone. In these conditions, blocking the effect of male hormones with anti-androgen medication should be accompanied with vigorous evaluation for the causes of hormonal imbalance.

Hair transplant surgery provides great results for women with hair loss when properly indicated. It is important to reiterate that many women with female pattern baldness are not good candidates for hair transplant. Again, this is because their donor hair area is also involved in the process of the baldness (the hair is also thinning out in that area). However, if the area of baldness is small and patient expectations are realistic, some women with less than perfect donor hair can also see improvement with hair transplant. A thorough consultation and examination with a hair restoration surgeon who is an expert in female hair loss provides the best and most successful path.

## FEMALE HAIRLINE LOWERING

Female hairline lowering can easily be accomplished thanks to FUE or FUT hair transplant. Some women have a high hairline because of genetics, male patterned hair loss or other surgical procedures. A hair transplant is an effective way to permanently reshape or reposition a female hairline from a masculine, or receded one, to a more feminine and attractive hairline.

### Hairline Lowering by Hair Transplant

- A hairline can be lowered by transplanting healthy follicles into the new hairline location. Special attention should be given to the direction and distribution of the transplanted hair. Every hair should be placed considering the direction, curvature and distribution of native hair in the area. Designing a new hairline for a woman who never had a natural hairline is a meticulous process. A hairline should be designed while considering the proportions of the entire face. A natural hairline makes the face more proportional and brings balance and harmony to the face.
- Some patients may bring pictures of women with perfect hairlines. If the structure of the face is similar, it is possible to recreate these hairlines. At times, the doctor may recommend a different hairline after examining the other components of the face and determining which hairline looks better

on you. Women who undergo a hairline lowering procedure, due to patterned baldness or previous facial procedures that may cause an elevated hairline, may decide to make their hairline more attractive than what they originally had. Adding lateral humps (protrusion of hairline on the sides) and widow's peak (forward advancement of the center of the hairline) adds character and charm to the faces of some women while helping to better frame their faces.

- Both FUE and FUT can be used to harvest hair from the donor area for hair lowering procedures. FUE is the procedure of choice for women who don't want any pain after the procedure or a scar on the back of their head.

- One hair transplant procedure is usually enough to define the new hairline and establish it in a new location. Some women may need another hair transplant procedure six month after the first one for better hairline definition. Women with coarse hair get better density and fullness with one procedure. If the hair shaft is fine, another procedure may be needed to add density and create a more solid hairline. If a second procedure is needed, it should be performed six months after the initial hair transplant.

- **Alternative Procedure**
  Surgical hairline lowering removes a strip of skin from the upper portion of the forehead and, by doing that, lowers the hairline. This surgical procedure has a quick effect and, unlike hair transplant results, the lowered hairline might be noticed immediately after the procedure. A few disadvantages of surgical hairline lowering are that the scar will be noted in front of the hairline and also the presence of a linear and unnatural hairline. Some patients may need a small hair transplant procedure to break down the straight line of the

hairline and to hide the linear scar in front by putting a few hair follicles in the front of their surgical scar.

- **What to Expect after Hair Transplant for Hairline Lowering**
Initial healing after a hair transplant takes about 3-5 days. Some redness and scabbing might be present for the first 5 days. The surgeon will usually provide a post-op kit that includes a special shampoo and sponge that can be used at home after your procedure. There might be some swelling and redness on the transplanted area and forehead. Many women choose to wear their bangs over the transplanted area or they may choose to wear a hat to cover the transplanted areas for the first few days.

- **When to Expect Results**
Hair transplant results can be seen after the first three months but it takes a few more months for the new hair to grow longer. The results of a hair restoration procedure to lower the hairline follow the typical pattern of other hair transplant procedures. The results are usually seen 8 to 12 months from the time of the procedure. The full appearance of the new hair is seen when the hair is long enough and can be combed and styled.

# HAIR RESTORATION PROCEDURE

## A BRIEF HISTORY

Baldness has been around for as long as people have had hair. Ancient archeological records suggest that even in the lofty cultures of grandeur, ancient Egypt and the more modern Roman Empire, hair loss was something to hide. Elaborate headpieces and wigs were used by the noble classes of these civilizations to represent an eternal youthful appearance.

Nearly two centuries ago in Wurzburg, Germany the first written record of medical hair restoration was documented. A medical student, Diffenbach, reported on an experimental surgery in which he assisted his mentor Professor Dom Unger. These surgeries were conducted on animals and humans. Their reports indicated a successful transplantation of hair from one area of the scalp to another. In the following decades, there was little evidence to support that any surgeons utilized Unger's technique to treat androgenic alopecia (genetically inherited baldness.)

It was in the late nineteenth century that hair-bearing skin flaps and grafts were first adapted in the treatment of traumatic alopecia i.e. baldness caused by burns or other types of severe physical injury. In this period, "traveling medicine men" peddled homemade remedies touted as a cure for baldness. These concoctions were supposed to be drunk or rubbed on the scalp. News publications of that time also touted nostrums that were a "single cure all" for conditions ranging from cancer to baldness.

## HAIR RESTORATION SURGERY ENTERS MEDICAL MAINSTREAM

It was during the Great Depression of the 1930's that the first modern surgical techniques of hair transplantation were developed. In the year 1939, a Japanese dermatologist, Dr. S. Okuda, reported the correction of hair loss by transplanting hair-bearing skin on 200 patients. He utilized his techniques to correct hair loss on the scalp, eyebrows and the upper lip. The rest of the world did not become fully aware of these advancements and techniques until after World War II. Successful hair transplantations to areas of the body besides the scalp were also reported by Japanese surgeons throughout the 1940's and 1950's. The first reports in the United States to treat Androgenic alopecia were not until 1959. The techniques used were remarkably similar to those discovered by Dr. Okuda nearly three decades before.

## THE INNOVATION OF MODERN HAIR TRANSPLANTS

It was at this time that Norman Orentreich, MD pioneered the shaping of modern hair restoration. He presented a paper detailing the physiologic basis for successful hair transplantation based on the concept of "donor dominance" and "recipient dominance." He successfully verified his treatment for hereditary baldness by demonstrating that the growth characteristics of hair from the donor site would dominate when transplanted to a recipient (bald or balding) area. These principles, known as "Donor Dominance", established that hair could be transplanted from the bald resistant donor areas to the balding areas and continue to grow for a lifetime. This laid the foundation for modern hair transplantation. Orentreich's discovery was a landmark disproving previous theory on the cause of baldness and is credited for heralding modern hair restoration. Over the next two decades, hair restoration through hair transplants continuously gained in popularity even though the results were notably unusual.

## MICROGRAFTING COMES INTO VOGUE

### The Advent of Mini/Micro Grafts

The 1980's marked another watershed event: the development of micrografting or punch grafts. This change rapidly evolved into even more refined donor grafts. A good example is the development of the strip method of obtaining donor hair from the back of the head. The strip would then be excised into mini-grafts containing 4 to 8 hairs. Hair restoration surgeons were then better able to create the fullness and density desired in the recipient (balding) areas.

The artistry of some physicians began to take shape, using even smaller mini-grafts of one, two, and three to create a refined feathered hairline. This advancement was significant because early grafts often yielded a brush or 'doll like' stiff appearance to the hair. Rather than dozens of grafts, the new surgeries now transplanted several hundred grafts from the donor area to the recipient areas.

Throughout the next two decades, micrografting techniques in hair transplants continued to evolve and be refined by hair restoration surgeons. Through the use of high powered magnification, physicians performed very detailed labor-intensive surgeries. Utilizing naturally occurring "follicular unit groupings" of 1 – 4 hairs, the number of grafts being transplanted grew. The steady forward march of these innovations continued to increase the popularity of hair transplant surgery among hair loss sufferers.

Presently, FUT hair transplants are the optimum standard performed by the world's best hair transplant surgeons. Relocating hair as it naturally grows has brought hair restoration to an exceptional level of acceptance in medical cosmetic surgery. These ultra-refined follicular unit procedures enable patients to enjoy results that are positively life changing.

### 21st Century Hair Restoration

In the 21st century, the tremendous advances in microsurgical hair replacement techniques have led to an increase in its popularity and effectiveness. Men and women, who suffer a loss of self-image from hair loss, benefit from hair restoration methods and procedures that help to create natural looking hair. Today's hair restoration procedures are referred to as Follicular Unit Transplants (FUT.) There are two forms of this surgery that will be discussed in detail further in this chapter: Strip Method procedure and Follicular Unit Extraction

(FUE) procedure. Suffice it to say, if done right, both these procedures offer natural results to resolving androgenic alopecia or what is commonly known as pattern baldness.

## THE NEW ART & SCIENCE OF HAIR RESTO RATION

### *Follicular Unit Transplant (FUT)*

The days of artificial looking hair plugs used in hair restoration procedures are gone. Strident advancements in the science and art of hair transplantation surgery are taking place. Follicular Unit Transplant (FUT) is the modern state of the art standard in hair restoration. Highly successful hair restoration procedures provide patients with remarkably natural looking results. This is because FUT involves a transplanting of the patient's own hair.

The beauty of FUT is that hair graft units are transplanted in their natural grouping from the donor scalp areas to the recipient (balding) areas. Follicular units consist of one to four terminal hair follicles. In addition to the normal hair follicles, each follicular unit consists of sebaceous (oil) glands, a small muscle, tiny nerves and small blood vessels. Every follicular unit is covered by the surrounding sheath primarily made of collagen protein.

A follicular unit is not only an anatomic unit but also a physiologic one. Preserving other important structures in a follicular unit ensures that each hair functions normally and looks natural. This is the basis for modern hair transplants where natural and undetectable results are expected with every hair transplant surgery

*Types of FUT Transplant*

There are two types of follicular unit hair transplant procedures each with their own unique benefits and disadvantages depending on the needs of the patient. The key difference in these procedures is the way in which donor hair from the patient is harvested from the permanent zone (the back and sides of the scalp). The two types of FUT hair restoration procedures are:

1. **The Strip Method**
   This more traditional method was the most common hair transplant procedure for many years. A strip is taken from the permanent zone of the scalp and then the surgical wound is closed. The follicular units are then harvested from the strip of scalp. The harvested grafts are then put into recipient incisions made by the surgeon in the balding and/or thinning areas of the scalp.

2. **Follicular Unit Extraction (FUE)**
   This method is currently the most common hair transplant procedure worldwide. It involves having the follicular units removed from the permanent zone individually. The individually harvested grafts are then placed into the recipient areas of the scalp.

*FUT Procedure*

FUT hair transplant procedures should only be performed by a medical doctor who is a hair transplant surgeon. The surgeon must be assisted by highly skilled medical technicians. Your hair transplant surgeon and his skilled medical team will perform a hair restoration procedure which should last for around 4 to 10 hours.

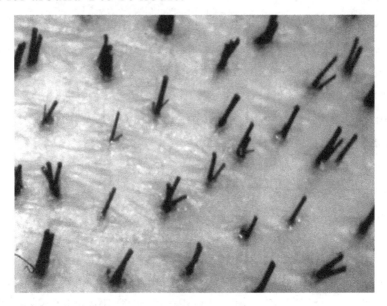

*FU, Magnified follicular units on scalp illustrating the natural grouping of hair.*

Hair transplant surgery results have been significantly improved through the introduction of stereoscopic microscopes and advanced methods of follicular extraction that are used in harvesting hair follicular units for implantation (grafts). Studies demonstrate that only increased magnification while performing the procedure can greatly improve the quality of the grafts and maximize the yield of intact healthy hair.

## BENEFITS OF HARVESTING NATURAL FOLLICULAR UNITS

- The ability to harvest follicular units more precisely in natural groupings reduces scarring at recipient sites in most patients.
- It creates less damage to follicles during harvesting (transaction) and therefore a maximum number of

grafts are available for transplantation.

- Hair grafts can be placed closer together in a natural pattern creating a look of greater density.

Natural looking hairlines are created through physician skill and ability to control direction of hair growth.

## THE NATURAL RESULTS

Follicular unit hair transplant surgery is the gold standard hair transplant procedure because of its functionality and natural look. The natural look obtained in hair restoration is primarily due to the fact that the surgeon is able to skillfully control the direction of the follicular grafts. Hair transplant surgeons can place follicular units artfully in the precise natural direction and with balanced distribution.

However, the old techniques of micrograft, mini-graft or plugs left surgeons little to no control on the distribution and direction of each follicular unit. The way the hair units are located in the donor area dictated their final direction after the hair transplant.

Today's male and female hair transplant patients are able to achieve a final surgical result that enhances their self-image and one that is mostly undetectable.

# BEFORE AND AFTER HAIR TRANSPLANT SURGERY

## *One Day Before Surgery*

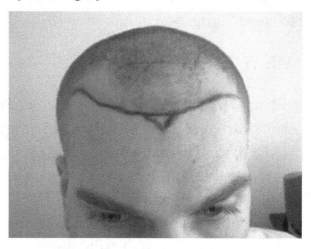

*Dr. Mohebi designs a new, natural hairline to create a non-balding appearance.*

## *Ten Days Following Surgery*

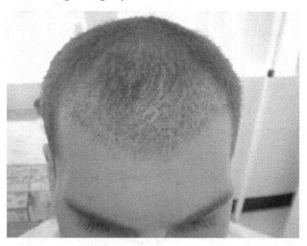

*The staples are removed at this phase. Some or all implanted hair will fall out and the hair follicles go to resting (telogen) phase. However, the implanted follicles will begin growing normal hair in a few months.*

61

## *Three Months after Hair Transplant Surgery*

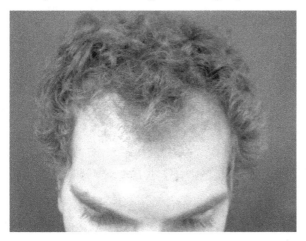

*Gradual growth of hair follicles is seen at this phase. The follicles will be all out growing by six months after a hair transplant surgery. However, it may take over twelve months until you can see them in their best shape and size.*

## **Eight Months after Hair Transplant Surgery**

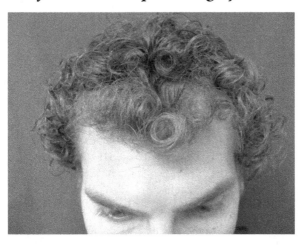

*All transplanted hair has grown by this time. Hair shafts may not be at their final length and pigmentation yet. Patients may need 10 to 18 months from the time of their surgery to be able to see the final result based upon the quality of transplanted hair and the style of their hair.*

## IS HAIR TRANSPLANT SURGERY FOR ME?

Whether or not you need a hair transplant surgery has to do with many different questions that an experienced hair transplant surgeon can easily answer by evaluating your scalp on both the balding and donor areas. It also may have to do with your family pattern and age of patterned hair loss presentation.

## AGE OF HAIR TRANSPLANTATION

### *Is there an age limit to having hair transplant surgery?*

Unlike what was suggested in the past, there is no age limit for having a hair transplant surgery as long as pros and cons of the procedure have been carefully evaluated by an experienced doctor. Many surgeons recommend that young men wait until they are older (above early 20s). This is because it is the age when most men's hairlines have matured and better enables the doctor to predict the advancement of the individual's pattern of baldness. Microscopic evaluation of the hair loss area can help a doctor predict where the patients are heading in the future. In addition to that, availability of new, effective hair loss medications has made it unnecessary for us to wait until the patient is completely showing more advanced stages of hair loss. Today, hair loss patients can choose to have a hair transplant performed at an earlier age. This is especially important now that we know about the adverse psychological effects of hair loss on hair loss patients.

## MOST MEN ARE CANDIDATES FOR HAIR TRANSPLANT

Androgenic alopecia or male pattern baldness (MPB) is the most frequent cause of hair loss in men. MPB can begin in early adolescence for some young men and can be a significant source of stress for them. The risk of MPB increases with age. It is estimated that more than fifty percent of men over fifty years of age have some degree of hair loss. It is this type of hair loss that is readily mitigated through hair restoration surgery. According to research, this type of hair loss affects more than thirty million men in the United States alone. It is these genetic factors that make most men with patterned baldness proper candidates for hair transplant surgery.

## ONLY SOME WOMEN ARE CANDIDATES

Why are only some women candidates for hair transplant surgery? Women can also have androgenic alopecia which is the form of pattern baldness like men. In many ways, this makes hair loss in women much more devastating.

## MEDICATIONS PRIOR TO HAIR TRANSPLANT

A hair restoration surgeon's consultation and evaluation should ascertain that there is no underlying cause of hair loss other than pattern baldness from androgenic alopecia. If hair loss is caused from other conditions such as Telogen Effluvium that can occur post-pregnancy, the condition must be treated first. It can occur after other types of stresses in men or women. This and other types of hair loss conditions should be treated prior to moving forward with a hair restoration surgery.

## BODY DYSMORPHIC SYNDROME

Body Dysmorphic Syndrome is a condition characterized by excessive preoccupation with an imaginary or minor bodily defect. In some people, the condition is severe enough to cause a decline in the patient's social, occupational or educational functioning. This is seen with some patients who believe they are suffering from hair loss when a complete medical evaluation demonstrates that they are not. It is very important that a hair transplant doctor evaluates the patient to confirm the diagnosis and to ascertain the need for a hair transplant surgery.

## MEN

The majority of male hair loss sufferers are men. As we said before, Male Pattern Baldness (MPB) is by far the primary cause of hair loss in men. By the age of fifty, more than fifty percent of men have noticeable hair loss and the percentage increases dramatically with each passing decade. By the age of seventy years, nearly ninety percent of men experience noticeable hair loss from androgenic alopecia. This hereditary genetic factor makes many men great candidates to enjoy the natural benefits of hair restoration. Hair transplant surgery is becoming the preferable choice for many.

The donor hair for men is taken from areas that are naturally resistant to MPB in most cases. Donor hair primarily resides at the back and, sometimes, the sides of the head. These hairs, when transplanted to balding areas, most often thrive and provide the patient with satisfying results.

## WOMEN

Hair loss in women is in many ways different than in men. For this reason, a few women suffering from hair loss find hair transplant to be the best option. Women typically lose hair at a more diffused pattern all over the scalp. This is often described as thinning and not balding by female hair loss sufferers. However, there are a significant number of women who inherit pattern baldness. These women can take advantage of the advancements in hair transplant surgery and technology to achieve a wonderful solution to their hair loss.

## EVALUATION BEFORE HAIR TRANSPLANT

A thorough evaluation including scalp and hair microscopic assessment, also known as the miniaturization study, should be part of an initial evaluation for every hair loss patient. Obtaining personal family history regarding baldness is critical in making the proper diagnosis. A detailed history should be taken that includes the time, speed and quality of hair loss and its association with other medical, physical or emotional factors.

A history of past and current medical problems is particularly useful in women with female pattern baldness because it helps discover any treatable disorder that may have caused or accelerated the process of hair loss. Some of the most common disorders are iron deficiency, thyroid disorders, autoimmune diseases such as lupus, hormonal imbalances such as an increase in male hormone and altered estrogen or progesterone levels. Some medications could cause hair loss in both men and women in which case, a more detailed history of medication use would be obtained.

Miniaturization study or recording the hair caliber changes on a microscopic level is used to diagnose most common hair loss patterns. Microscopic evaluation is also used to predict future hair loss. The initial evaluation includes measurements of donor quality and scalp laxity. Those two factors are key to patients who undergo a hair transplant procedure.

The kind of results a person should expect after hair transplant surgery has to do with many factors. It is mostly related to the characteristics of the hair in the donor area. These characteristics include thicker hair vs. thinner hair, wavy vs. straight and minimum contrast of hair color with the skin tone. Less contrast means less visibility of the scalp and less appearance of baldness.

An examination is important because it helps the doctor to determine a person's qualifications for hair transplantation and to estimate the number of grafts needed.

## HOW DOES A HAIR TRANSPLANT WORK?

Hair restoration through hair transplant surgery is the only natural permanent solution for androgenic alopecia. Hair on the back and sides of the head is referred to as the permanent zone. It is because the hair in those areas is genetically resistant to baldness. The permanent zone is also known as the donor area. Hair from donor area is transplanted to the bald areas (recipient area) for hair restoration.

This success of using genetically resistant hair from a permanent zone is the reason why the hair transplant surgery trend has been on the rise in the last few decades. This procedure is also becoming more popular among women. Hair transplantation is being used for eyebrow hair loss or to restore hair on any other part of the body that a patient desires.

Hair restoration can also be used for treatment of hair loss due to physical injuries including burns, congenital deformities and surgical scars that cause hair loss.

Today, there is only one natural solution to hair loss. That is hair restoration through hair transplant surgery. These procedures for eliminating hair loss involve the surgical removal of donor hair from the back and/or sides of the scalp to the thinning and balding areas. Today's microscopic hair transplant surgery is so refined that it is mostly undetectable.

Hair is harvested from the donor area in its natural grouping of one to four hairs. These groupings are called follicular units. Hair transplant surgeons make artful incisions into the recipient (balding) area(s.) The results of modern hair restoration are highly successful and natural because it is the persons own hair restored in a natural realistic pattern.

Hair restoration surgery has been the preferred choice of treatment for male patterned baldness (MPB). The tremendous recent advances contribute to the growth of hair transplantation for others including female pattern baldness (FPB), eyebrow hair loss or restoring hair on any part of the body.

It is important for people to know that the surgical procedures used in hair restoration must be performed by a medical doctor who specializes in performing hair transplant surgery.

## STRIP METHOD HAIR TRANSPLANT

The strip method procedure was the most widely performed hair transplant procedure in hair restoration for men and women for many years. You will also hear this mentioned as follicular unit transplantation (FUT). In fact, the strip method is only one specific form of FUT. Strip method is a good choice of hair restoration for many people because the individual hair follicles stay intact and they are very rarely damaged by this technique. This is because the natural follicular units remain intact throughout harvesting and implanting. The follicular units contain 1 to 4 hairs per follicular unit.

When performing the strip method procedure, the hair transplant surgeon uses microscopes allowing for a refined dissection of each hair follicle. The lack of heat generated by these microscopes further preserves the integrity of the harvested follicular units. Each unit is preserved in a special temperature-controlled solution while the doctor designs the recipient sites.

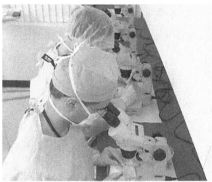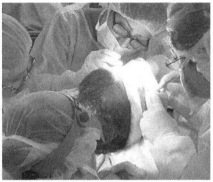

*Follicular Unit dissection and placement of grafts*

# CRITICAL FACTORS IN STRIP HAIR TRANS-PLANTATION

In medical procedures, there are numerous factors that lead to a successful outcome. The qualifications, knowledge and experience of the surgical team provide hair restoration patients with a lifelong attractive natural result. These critical factors include:

- Correct donor extraction and wound care
- Excellence in follicular unit dissection
- Quality control in graft preparation
- Graft hydration and storage
- Age appropriate, natural hairline design
- Recipient site creation using proper angulations, direction and arrangement
- Careful placement of grafts with the proper technique
- Diligent post-surgical follow up at appropriate intervals

Dissecting the strip into grafts is key to maximizing the number of available donor follicular units and optimizing all other results in a patient's hair transplant. A strip is dissected into smaller pieces called slivers (see images). Next, the slivers are dissected into follicular units or grafts. A well-trained team ensures that grafts are not wasted due to poor technique. Proper dissection results in a high level of hair growth after hair transplantation.

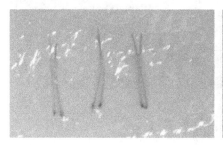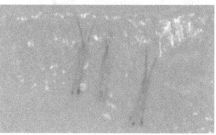

*Double hair and triple hair FUT samples.*

# FOLLICULAR UNIT EXTRACTION (FUE)

### What is FUE?

Follicular Unit Extraction (FUE) is the method of harvesting hair grafts directly and individually from the patient donor area. This process of collecting hair units was first introduced by Dr. Woods in Australia. Other hair transplant doctors further standardized it.

Follicular Unit Extraction (FUE) may also be called Follicular Isolation Technique (FIT). One of the advantages of FUE is that patients will not have a linear scar or pain and tightness on the donor area of the scalp. There is no need to remove a strip of skin from the donor area in FUE hair transplantation. Patients usually do not experience donor complications seen with the strip technique such as pain and discomfort or wound closure problems in donor area after hair transplant. There is no need for staple or suture removal after the procedure and there will not be a linear scar in the donor area.

## *The History of FUE*

Japanese doctors are known to be the first to describe how skin containing hair could be moved from one area to the other while keeping its ability to grow hair. They performed the initial successful transplantation of hair follicles in order to treat scar and burn patients in the 1930s by transplanting small pieces of skin to those areas. Dr. Norman Orentreich, a dermatologist in New York City, demonstrated the theory of donor dominance in 1959. He proved that plugs of skin, with hair follicles from the back of the scalp, can continue growing hair after being implanted into balding areas. He has since performed the initial plug transplantation in America. Those initial plug surgeries are the ancestors of the current FUE transplantation.

Dr. Woods from Australia was the first doctor who harvested single follicular units using smaller punch devices. His smaller size punches allowed transplantation of the individual follicular units without removing a plug or a strip of skin. He presented his surgical technique of using 1mm punch in 1995. Despite the novelty of his technique, his attempt to publish this method in medical journals was not successful.

Drs. Rassman and Bernstein were the first physicians who jointly published the methodology of harvesting hair follicles, as we call them Follicular Unit Extraction, or FUE, in 2002. FUE method of removing individual follicular units was first performed with larger punches (larger than 1mm). In recent years, more modernized methods and the use of smaller punches were introduced to the field of hair restoration. The non-invasive nature of FUE procedures and the possibility of eliminating the linear scar has made it a very popular method of hair transplantation in the last few years. Currently, there are several motorized devices such as suction assisted harvesting techniques and robotic arm on the market for harvesting follicles with FUE method.

### FUE versus Strip Hair Transplant

FUE transplant techniques have been improved tremendously in the last decade. However, both FUE and strip hair transplants are still being used and they each have their advantages and disadvantages. The option of choosing one method versus the other should be evaluated after a thorough examination of the hair loss situation by a hair transplant surgeon.

Choosing FUE transplant versus strip method involves several factors including the total number of permanent donor hair in relation to the number of hairs that the person may require during life. The patient should make the final decision about the type of hair transplantation based on factors such as the extent of hair loss, quality of donor hair and the patient's expectations. Here we will review the most common advantages of each technique:

### FUE Transplant Advantages

- It does not leave a linear scar on the donor area so the patient can choose to keep hair on the back of their head very short or even shaved
- There is very minimal pain and discomfort after FUE transplant.
- There is a minimal chance of donor complications such as wound necrosis or temporary hair loss after hair transplant (shock loss) in donor area after FUE procedures

- Total evenness of hair density could be only achieved with an FUE procedure. That means the procedure not only adds hair to the balding areas but it can reduce the high density of the donor zone to minimize the contrast between the two areas. Minimizing the contrast can always make the recipient look less bald.

## Strip Transplant Advantages
- A higher number of grafts can be harvested in one procedure in strip transplants. Today we can easily transplant over 2500 grafts in most patients in their first hair transplant procedure with the strip method.
- Strip hair transplant is generally more affordable than FUE transplants in most practices due to its labor intensity
- No need to shave the donor area in strip method. Of course, this problem could be avoided in FUE procedures now with Celebrity or Layer Shaving techniques.

It is advisable that every hair loss patient choose their hair transplantation option only after reviewing all the pros and cons of strip versus FUE hair transplant methods. It is also important for hair transplant surgeons to consider individual hair characteristics, demand for hair and the patient's personal goals when selecting the right hair transplant procedure.

## Who is a Good Candidate for FUE?
FUE can be recommended for almost anyone. People who want to have the option to shave their head or wear their hair very short may have no other options. Although the linear scar caused by strip could be minimized by a variety of techniques of wound closure, there is still no way to guarantee the line of scar will not be visible if the patient chooses to shave

his head.

People who only need a small number of grafts to restore limited areas of the scalp are among those who may want to choose the FUE procedure.

Another group of patients who may want to choose FUE are those who have had a bad experience in the past with complications of a strip procedure or those that have significant scarring which makes the removal of more follicles through strip impossible.

### Different Methods of FUE

FUE devices and methods have been transformed considerably in the last two decades. Manual methods, which are still in use by some clinics, have been refined with more perfected punches. There are a variety of sharp and dull punches and a combination of them. Motorized methods of FUE harvesting have been around for many years. They include rotating versus oscillating that could be utilized with sharp versus dull punches.

Some motorized FUE devices are equipped with a suction mechanism to extract grafts after they are punched from the scalp. There have been controversies on the benefits of adding suction to the FUE machines because of the potential negative effect of the suction on the viability of the grafts.

Finally, Robotic Hair Restoration is another innovative device in the field of hair restoration. The robot allows detection of the follicular units and its topography with several cameras. The images from the cameras can detect the location, distribution, and the angulation of the follicular grafts. The robotic arm has been able to increase the speed of graft extraction and more importantly to minimize the exhaustion of the surgeon during a FUE hair transplant. Despite the advantages of robotic hair restoration systems, there are still some disadvantages to it such as the size of the punches are still relatively large in comparison to what is used in other methods of FUE. The high price of the device is another disadvantage sometimes totaling up to the whole price of the cost of a hair transplant.

## FUE Complications

FUE hair transplant like any other surgical procedure has its complications. Here are some of the common complications of a FUE transplant:

- **Transection of hair follicles:**

  The most common complication of the FUE procedure, especially if it is not done in the right hands or with the proper technique, is the high rate of transection. Transection is the dissection of the grafts somewhere along its length that prevents extraction of an intact follicle. Transection rate may be higher with some devices in comparison to others. It may also be higher in wavy hairs. It seems that many of the transected grafts will grow in the donor area.

- **Hypopigmentation:**

  This is when the spots of the harvested FUE grafts look lighter than the neighboring areas. This phenomenon was more common in the past when larger sizes of punches were used. As the FUE punches get smaller, the risk of hypopigmentation is reduced. This complication may only be seen when the patient keeps his/ her hair very short or shaves his/ her head. This condition is usually not seen as much when smaller size punches are used. Hypopigmentation could be treated with Scalp Micropigmentation (SMP) which adds dermal pigments that resemble hair and minimize the visibility of the lighter areas.

- **Folliculitis/Cyst formation:**

  This condition can be seen in both strip and FUE method when the hair follicle in the donor or recipient area becomes inflamed. This might be due to the closure of the exit pores of the oil glands that naturally occur around hair (sebaceous glands). Folliculitis may look like atypical facial acne and is usually dissolved spontaneously without any treatment. If it persists, the doctor can incise and drain the pimples in the office.

- **Ingrown hair:**

  Ingrown hair might be seen occasionally in the donor area especially when the follicular transection rate is higher than normal. The lesions occasionally require incision and removal of the trapped hair that can be done easily in a doctor's office.

## HOW TO GET READY FOR YOUR FUE PROCEDURE

Once the final decision is made to undergo Follicular Unit Extraction (FUE), there are a few easy steps you need to follow to prepare for your procedure.

In general, preparation for FUE begins a few days before the procedure.

## *Five to Ten Days before FUE:*

- **Medical problems** – If you have any ongoing medical issues or concerns, please discuss your upcoming hair transplant procedure with your primary care doctor as soon as possible so your doctor can make sure you are cleared for the surgery.
- **Medications** – Once you are cleared by your primary care physician, stop taking medications that may increase the chances of bleeding during surgery. Common medications that are held for this surgery include:
  1. **Antiplatelet** medications (Aspirin, Plavix and Pradaxa) due to an increased risk of bleeding during and after the procedure
  2. **Anti-inflammatory** medications (ibuprofen aka Motrin or Advil and naproxen aka Aleve)
  3. **Anticoagulation** medications (warfarin aka Coumadin) and all of the newer anticoagulation medications such as Xarelto.
  4. Some **over-the-counter** products can also have an anticoagulation effect and they should be avoided before most surgical procedures (Fish oil, vitamin E, Omega 3, St Johns Wart, Gingko)
- **Communicate with your doctor** – Please let your hair transplant doctor know, as soon as possible, if you have any **new medical conditions** or if you are taking any **new medications** since your initial consultation appointment. This is necessary so the doctor can choose medications that will not interact with your existing medications during surgery. If you are not sure about whether to hold a specific medication before surgery, please call your doctor's office to inquire.

### *Three Days before FUE:*

- **Stop smoking** – It is best to stop smoking at least three to five days before your FUE procedure. Smoking causes blood vessels to constrict which results in a decreased blood flow to the scalp. In addition, you should also refrain from smoking during the first five days after your procedure.

### *Two Days before Surgery:*

- Scalp to Scalp – No special hair preparation is necessary since the hair on the donor area will be trimmed with a clipper to the length of 1mm on the day of surgery. The only exception to this is non-shaven or celebrity FUE transplantation in which the hair is kept long. This short trim allows for the best access to, and easy removal and placement of, grafts. At times, the entire scalp will be trimmed to make it easier to harvest and place the grafts but, in some cases, hair trimming can be minimized to the donor area. An alternative method is to shave the donor area in layers, AKA layer shaving, if you have hair that is long enough where the areas between the shaved bands can provide enough hair to cover the shaved areas. Please don't get a short haircut before your procedure if you are considering this option.
- Beard to Scalp – This involves a razor shave of the beard/upper neck 2 days before your procedure. Shaving 2 days prior allows the surgeon, on the day of surgery, to better differentiate the hairs in the anagen stage (growth phase) vs. the hairs in the resting telogen phase. The hairs in the growth phase will grow in those 2 days to a length of approximately 1mm while those in the resting phase are somewhat dormant and will not grow at the same rate. Hair exhibiting active growth

will be harvested while hairs in the resting telogen phase will not be harvested and left untouched.

- Body to Scalp – Much like beard to scalp, patients are asked to razor shave the body areas within the donor sites two days prior to the procedure.
- Scalp to Eyebrow – A small procedure where any necessary trimming is done at the time of surgery.
- Celebrity FUE – This is a very popular choice for patients who wish to have FUE performed in a virtually undetectable manner. There is no prior hair preparation involved as limited individual trimming is done during the procedure. You need to keep your hair long and the hairs used in the transplant are trimmed one by one.

*Day of Procedure:*
- **Dress Comfortably** – You will want to be comfortable during the FUE procedure since it may range from five to ten hours depending on the number of grafts you receive. Wear a shirt that can easily be unbuttoned from the front. Don't wear a shirt that needs to be pulled over your head to prevent the likelihood of contacting and dislodging the grafts.
- **Wash Your Hair** – Shower and wash your hair in the morning prior to arriving at our office. Using your regular shampoo is fine but do not apply products such as mouse, hairspray or gel to your hair the morning of your procedure.
- **Arranging for Post-Op** – You will most likely receive sedatives at the beginning, or during, the procedure to keep you relaxed. Please arrange post-op transportation as you will be unable to drive due to the sedation used during your procedure.

# CELEBRITY FUE HAIR RESTORATION

Celebrity FUE is a hair transplant procedure that has grown in popularity in recent years among celebrities and others who wish to keep their hair transplant anonymous. This out-patient procedure involves minimal post-surgical downtime and little to no detectability. This novel hair restoration technique was pioneered and perfected by Dr. Parsa Mohebi.

## *Advantages*
The benefits of Celebrity FUE include:
- Little to no pain or discomfort during, and after, the procedure
- No need to shave the donor or recipient area
- No visible scars

Its minimal downtime allows patients to continue working without disruption. This procedure is an excellent choice for patients who wish to keep their hair transplant as discreet as possible by reducing the typical post-operative appearance.

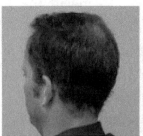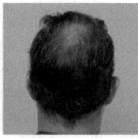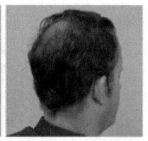

*Immediately After a Celebrity FUE Transplant – No Shaving – No Scarring*

## *Limitations*
The one disadvantage of Celebrity FUE transplantation is the limited number of grafts that can be transplanted per session. People with higher stages of hair loss, or those that require a larger number of grafts, may need more than one day to har-

vest the required number of grafts.

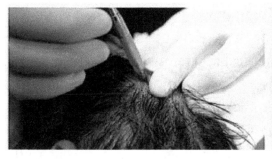 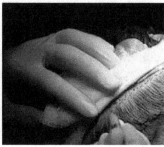

*The Celebrity FUE technique allows patients to keep their hair long during their procedure*

## HAIR TRANSPLANT REPAIR

Hair transplant has evolved over the last few decades. Many patients who had a hair restoration using outdated techniques are reluctant to seek a second hair transplant, or revision hair transplant, due to a less than ideal experience the first time. The fear of an unknown outcome, or the rehashing of a perceived unpleasant prior hair transplant experience, is enough to lead clients to shy away from a revision hair transplant.

The advent of newer techniques has made potential candidates more likely to benefit from the latest techniques that make hair transplants virtually undetectable.

This is promising news for individuals who previously underwent a hair transplant using outdated methods such as hair plugs or mini/ micro grafts. A corrective procedure using the latest techniques of FUE or FUT will improve the appearance of unsightly plugs. In most cases, a revision hair transplant can restore a more natural appearance to an otherwise unnatural look.

## *Pluggy Hairlines*

During its inception, hair transplantation hair plugs ranged in size from 2-10 mm. These plugs could move hair from the donor to balding areas of the scalp but they were unable to create a hairline with a natural appearance. In the early years, plug surgery hairlines were like tufts of isolated hair, amid an ocean of scalp, making transplanted hair obvious and unsightly. In the ensuing years, plug surgery improved with grafts decreasing in size to as small as 1-2 mm. These grafts were called minigrafts and micrografts and were considered a vast improvement over plugs. Despite being smaller grafts, the results were still detectable.

**Treatment of plugs** – Plug revision, and an improvement of the outward appearance of the surrounding scalp, can easily be achieved with the new FUE methods. By utilizing this method, two problems are addressed concurrently:

1. Plugs with 100% density of hair will be thinned out by removing some of the hair follicles thereby reducing the density.
2. Surrounding areas with 0% hair will receive the transplanted follicular units while creating a more natural grouping. This maneuvering of grafts will give greater density and can eliminate the "pluggy" appearance.

## *Hairline with Large Grafts*

The typical appearance of a native (non-transplanted) hairline is typically comprised of two rows of follicular units consisting of one single hair. Between the extraction and placement process, hairs are sorted and counted. If this step is skipped, and hairs are not properly selected before placement, there is a good chance grafts containing 2 or 3 hairs will be erroneously placed in the hairline and result in an unnatural look. This issue is particularly noticeable if the patient has coarse hair.

The proper method of designing and creating a natural hairline is only transplanting grafts with a single hair in the very front 0.5 to 1cm of the hairline. Singles are followed by grafts with 2 hairs to the rear and then grafts with 3 and 4 hairs. This natural order will give good density and bulk to the more posterior area, and beyond, while creating a natural transitional zone in the very front.

**Treatment of hairline with larger grafts** – Successful revision of detectable hairlines can easily be achieved based on the original location of the hairline:

1. If the hairline was originally placed higher than its natural location, a natural hairline can be created using only single hair grafts.
2. If the original transplanted hairline was placed too low, it is necessary to remove any grafts with 2 or 3 hairs and replace them with naturally occurring single hair grafts. A very common miscalculation of early transplants was the placement of grafts containing 2 or 3 hairs along the front row of the hairline. Thus, the presence of multi-hair grafts on the hairline is a dead giveaway of an older transplant.

**Unnatural hairline design**

Revision procedures are typically performed on older hair transplants. However, newly transplanted hair can appear noticeable due to poor design. In such cases, there is usually a mismatch with an age inappropriate hairline or a total disregard for the ethnicity of the patient. Hairlines are sometimes designed by inexperienced doctors who overlook the relationship of the hairline to the other landmarks of the face.

When designing the hairline, there are intentional micro and macro irregularities built into the design to prevent the hairline from having a "connect the dots with a straight line" appearance. The following occurrences, with respect to hairline design, may result in an unnatural hairline:

- **A juvenile hairline** – The average non-balding man undergoes a maturation of the hairline in most ethnicities. Thus, recreating a juvenile hairline on an aging man is not realistic. Expectations must be created with the goal of creating a mature and natural appearing hairline.

- **A linear/straight hairline** – A normal adult hairline should possess both macro-irregularity and micro-irregularity to form a natural looking hairline. Regrettably, some surgeons may try to make the hairline too perfect while forgetting the importance of these natural occurring irregularities. This is a common mistake in hair transplants performed by inexperienced practitioners. There is an easy solution! Simply adding inherent micro-irregularities is an easy fix and does not require many grafts.

- **Thin hairline** – Inadequate density along the hairline, and just beyond, typically results in an outcome that appears unnatural. This thinning might be unavoidable in patients who possess fine hair from the onset of the process. At this point in time, it is inconceivable to restore hair back to its original 100% density with only one hair transplant procedure. Patients with thick/coarse hair can expect a more solid hairline with only one hair transplant procedure. During the hairline planning stage, meticulous attention to detail is required to achieve a natural hairline. The placement of an adequate number of grafts to achieve optimal density, and strategic placement of the appropriately sized follicular units, is necessary.

- **Sex inappropriate hairline** – Hairlines of adult men are different than those of females. A perfectly natural masculine hairline would look completely unnatural and harsh on a woman and a feminine hairline would appear odd and dainty on a man. The corners on the hairline in adult men are usually receded in comparison to the hairline in the midfrontal area. A female hairline usually does not present a typical male recession of the corners. In contrast, a feminine hairline may be flat or curving downward. A very high hairline needs to be lowered through a hairline lowering transplant to produce a more attractive frame to the face. There are times when feminine hairlines have slight humps that can redefine and minimize the area of the visible forehead. Treatment of an unnatural hairline design is performed on a case by case basis. A hairline revision to create a more natural appearance can easily be accomplished in one or two procedures depending on what needs to be done. FUE hair transplantation can remove the unwanted hair follicles from the hairline and relocate them to a proper position elsewhere on the scalp.

## Scarring

Scarring left behind by older hair restoration methods is often seen in the donor or recipient areas. A widened linear donor scar is typically seen after FUT (follicular unit transplantation) performed via a strip procedure. The repair or revision of old donor scars can easily be done today using a variety of techniques such as trichophytic closure, FUE into the scar and SMP.

## *Incorrect hair orientation*

Native scalp hair follows a specific orientation in terms of direction and curvature. Therefore, when follicular unit grafts are implanted, the orientation in angulation and curvature must be adhered to in order to achieve natural looking results.

- Wrong angulation – Hair angles follow specific patterns in different areas of the scalp. The angles may change drastically in certain areas along the hairline. The angulation should be monitored and followed to create a perfectly natural hairline indistinguishable from a natural head of hair. Meticulous attention should be paid to the angle of the exiting native hair to achieve a completely natural result.

- Wrong curvature – Just like hair angles, the curvature of each hair differs from area to area on the scalp. Thoughtful vigilance to the curvature of each individual transplanted graft is important in creating an appearance that looks completely natural. Curvature of the hair shaft is particularly crucial in locations such as the temples, hairline and eyebrows. The angles of hair should be planned by a surgical team and revisited throughout the placing phase of the procedure. Upon final inspection, grafts may be rotated within their individual sites (if necessary) to adjust according to the natural hair curvature for each area.

**Treatment of incorrect hair orientation** – The best treatment for incorrect angulation and curvature of the hair is to prevent them. By using proper techniques, a hair transplant with an artistic flair can easily avoid these problems. In the event of such problems, ill-placed hair follicles should be removed via the FUE method and reimplanted to provide the proper angle and curvature.

# AFTER HAIR TRANSPLANTATION

## FIRST FEW DAYS AFTER HAIR TRANSPLANT

### Pain and discomfort

There may be some aching in the donor area for certain procedures such as strip hair transplant which starts within the first few hours after hair transplantation. FUE procedures are either painless or the pain is very minimal. Pain medicine is provided to alleviate discomfort during the first night. After the first night, the pain should be well controlled. Most patients do not need any medications for pain after the first day. If they are still experiencing pain during the second day, mild pain medications, such as Tylenol, are normally enough to bring more comfortable results.

### Swelling

Swelling is very common during the first four days after hair restoration surgery. Some swelling around the transplanted area is expected. Swelling is due to the process of healing and may range from nonexistent to severe in which the subcutaneous fluid descends from the forehead area to around the eyes. Maximum swelling is generally seen in days 3 and 4 after hair transplantation. Some patients may need steroids to prevent swelling after their hair restoration. It is good to sleep in a semi-sitting position and keep the upper body elevated to help minimize the swelling or shorten its duration.

*Bruising*

Bruising or discoloration of skin around the transplanted area might be present for the first few days after the procedure. This may involve the recipient area and, at times, may extend to the forehead. Covering the transplanted area with a hat can hide the area of swelling but those with existing hair can use it to cover the bruised areas of the transplanted sites.

*Scabbing*

Scabbing is common during the first week or two after a hair transplant. The scabs should flake off within one week if the patient washes the transplanted areas properly. It is a good practice to bring patients back for the first day after hair transplantation to give them a hair wash and teach them how to wash their head for the first few days. A special shampoo and sponge is needed for proper washing of hair that may vary in different practices. We recommend washing transplanted areas twice a day for the first 4 days. Patients can go back to their routine hair wash after that time unless they continue to have scabbing. They need to continue washing their head twice a day as long as they still have scabbing in the area.

*Itching*

Itching is a common symptom in any type of wound healing. Hair transplantation is not an exception to that reality. Patients may feel itching on transplanted and donor areas for the first few days. This may extend to the second week after hair transplant. However, it should be mild and does not require any treatment for most patients. If itching is significant, then a prescription of a moisturizing cream or a mild steroid cream might be needed.

### Washing Hair After Hair Transplant
The first 4 days after surgery are most critical as hair transplant patients need to be extra careful about washing their hair (especially in the transplanted areas). There is a special "hair washing" appointment the day after surgery designed to show the patient how to properly wash while taking critical care of the transplanted areas. After 4 days, most people can return to a normal hair washing routine.

### Returning to Work After Hair Transplant
You can return to work as early as the day after hair restoration surgery for FUE procedures. However, if you had a strip procedure and your job requires any kind of lifting, bending, stretching, physical strain or touching chemicals, patient should take a few days off until the acute phase is over. Some patients may need to take days off only because they want to keep their hair transplant surgery confidential. In these types of cases, a patient can take 1 to 2 weeks off work. The first four days are the most critical in being extra careful to avoid any type of strain. After four days, the transplanted grafts are usually well settled and they cannot be dislodged.

### Physical Activities After Hair Transplant
No physical activity that can cause strain on the back of head, sutured or stapled area should be done. There are no limitations for mild exercises as long as the patient does not bend

his/her head aggressively or touch the transplanted area. Contact sports should be avoided for the first month for most patients who had a transplant surgery.

## ONE WEEK AFTER HAIR TRANSPLANT

### *Redness and Inflammation*

The inflammation and redness should be subsided at this time but a mild pinkish discoloration of the transplanted area may remain. This can be visible for a few weeks and could be comparable to sunburn (especially in patients with lighter skin).

### *Physical Activity*

It is okay to resume exercise more than two days after the hair transplant. In strip procedures, it is critical to be selective about the types of exercises done (such as not doing squats, bent rows, lifts, etc.) for the first four days after surgery. Always aim to keep your head elevated and upright when possible. Bending the head may increase the tension of the donor area in strip procedures and may increase the chance of stretching of the scar.

### *Itching*

Itching is still common during this time as the surgical areas will continue healing during the first few weeks.

## FOUR WEEKS AFTER PROCEDURE

### *Redness and Inflammation*

The inflammation should be subsided by this point in most patients. Transplanted hair generally falls out in the first two to three weeks and patients go back to where they were before hair transplantation at this point.

*Physical Activity*

Patients should be able to resume most physical activities they used to do before hair transplantation. The key is avoiding strain on the scar area if a strip, or FUT, hair transplant was performed. If an FUE procedure was performed, more intense exercises are permitted.

# 3 MONTHS AFTER SURGERY

*Appearance*

The appearance of the patient should be similar to the pre-transplanted time. Patients generally don't keep the newly transplanted hair and commonly lose the shaft of hairs while the follicles become part of the scalp and generate new hairs.

*Shock Loss*

This is the worst period after hair transplantation due to the fact that some patients may lose some of their native hair due to shock loss after their hair transplant. This happens when the bulk of the transplanted hair hasn't grown in yet. Some patients may feel like the bulk of their hair is lessening more than what it was before the hair transplant. This does happen at times until the next few months after hair transplant when the patients can see the newly transplanted hair along with regrowth from some of the hair that has gone through shock loss.

*New Growth*

Patients, who have complete baldness with no visible hair before hair transplant, should be able to see some very small hair in the transplanted area. Many people may not see any new hair begin to grow out before the first six months after the procedure.

### *Folliculitis*

Folliculitis or pimple shaped lesions may be noted in some patients at this time. They generally form because of the collection of sebum (oily secretions of the hair follicles). Folliculitis lesions usually drain spontaneously without any need for any interventions. If your folliculitis lesions number more than two or are painful, you need to see your surgeon to have those lesions drained for you. Drainage of folliculitis is generally simple and painless.

## 6 MONTHS AFTER SURGERY

### *Telogen Effluvium*

Telogen Effluvium is sudden, and usually, stress related hair loss which presents itself as general thinning throughout the scalp. Telogen Effluvium occurs after any severe and sudden stress. In Telogen Effluvium, a large number of hair follicles go to the sleep phase at once causing hair loss or thinning all over or in a large area of the scalp. In most cases the hair loss recovers spontaneously and completely. Telogen Effluvium can be seen in patients who are prone to male or female patterned baldness and stress could accelerate hair loss that may be not reversible due to underlying conditions. The most common form of Telogen Effluvium is seen after childbirth or pregnancy termination.

# ONE YEAR AFTER HAIR TRANSPLANT

## *Hair Growth*

The final results from the hair restoration should be obvious and noticeable at this stage. Most of the new hair will have grown to its normal thickness at this time. Although most patients may see most of their results at this time, more improvement in fullness and thickness should be expected up until 18 months from the hair transplant. The size of the donor scar will mature during the first year and should be at its final size at this time in patients who had the strip hair transplant procedure.

# AFTER THE FIRST YEAR

More fullness should be expected at this point through 18 months from the hair transplant. This case is especially true for patients who grow their hair long. Many patients at this time can see the final results and determine whether a second hair restoration procedure is necessary.

It is crucial to stay in touch with your hair transplant surgeon after your hair transplantation if you have any concerns or questions. We at Parsa Mohebi Hair Restoration usually see our patients after their hair transplant surgery for 4 standard follow-up visits.

# HAIR TRANSPLANT RESULTS

Most people experience the loss of the hair shaft in their newly transplanted hair grafts within the first few weeks. It may take 2-3 months for the patients to see the regrowth of the new hair. Occasionally, this can be up to 6 to 8 months. Full results of the hair transplant surgery can be seen 10-12 months after surgery in the majority of patients.

The results of a hair transplant with follicular unit transplantation should be undetectable if the procedure is done correctly with proper techniques and by a qualified hair transplant surgeon. Most patients report that even their hair stylists cannot tell that they had a hair transplant done. The ability to take follicular units with 1, 2, 3 or 4 hairs allows for the surgeon and medical team to place hair follicles into recipient sites in a natural and realistic direction and distribution. The undetectable natural, and permanent, results of modern hair transplants provide patients with results that truly uplift their self-image and esteem (Mohebi & Rassman, 2008).

This success can also change the results for patients who had hair transplants before the advent of FUT procedures. These older procedures with very detectable results can be repaired and restored with the skills of an experienced hair restoration surgeon.

## HAIR TRANSPLANT COMPLICATIONS

Hair transplant is generally a skin level surgery so its side effects are minimal and limited to the skin level. Here are the most common complications of a hair transplant surgery:

## PAIN AND DISCOMFORT

Pain is very mild or nonexistent after an FUE procedure. Patients may have pain after a strip hair transplant surgery on the donor site. That is where the surgical wound is closed with either sutures or staples. Tightness of the area can also be a problem in cases where a large number of grafts are removed. Patients generally do not have any pain in the recipient area after a hair transplant procedure. Pain is mostly seen after strip hair transplantation as we discussed before. Donor pain can be controlled by blocking the area right before the conclusion of the procedure with infiltration of a local anesthetic. The block that is obtained by infiltration of local anesthetic may wear off a few hours after the hair transplant. Many patients may need pain medication for the first night after the surgery. The pain usually subsides the following day but discomfort of the sutured or stapled area on the back may remain for several days. Mild over-the-counter pain medication is generally sufficient to alleviate the pain in the following days.

## SWELLING AND INFLAMMATION

Like any other skin surgery, hair transplantation may cause swelling or redness for the first few days. The difference is that hair transplant swelling is usually not seen immediately after the hair transplant. It starts to be noticeable at around days 2 and 3. The swelling typically reaches its peak on days 3 and 4 and subsides immediately after that. Sleeping in a semi-sitting position at 30 to 45 degrees for the first few nights can help minimize the swelling. Swelling can be severe and move down to the areas around the eyes but it cannot jeopardize the survival of the grafts. If you have a high risk of swelling based on your prior surgical history, you may need anti-inflammatory medications to minimize the redness and swelling after a hair transplant. Steroids could be prescribed by your hair transplant surgeon to be used before, or after, your procedure.

## SHOCK LOSS

Shock loss is losing hair in an area with active hair loss due to stress. Shock loss after hair transplants used to be more common. However, it has been proven that using finasteride (Propecia) can prevent shock loss considerably. Minoxidil may have a similar effect on minimizing shock loss in areas with active hair loss. This may be a consideration in some women who undergo a hair transplant.

We recommend starting patients who have high risk of shock loss on one of these medications a few days before hair transplant. The treatment should continue for at least 6 to 8 months after the procedure.

Shock loss can also be seen around the donor area. Donor wound shock loss is mostly seen in the patients who require a large number of grafts and the ones with a tight scalp. Hair loss around the donor area is more common among women due to the smaller proportions of their head circumference to the width of the strip.

Shock loss is a type of Telogen Effluvium in which a large number of hair follicles enter their resting phase at the same time. Growing hair follicles that are forced to enter a resting phase lose their hair shaft temporarily. This hair thinning may continue for a few months but it usually resolves completely without any need for treatment.

# FOLLICULITIS

Folliculitis is a pimple-like skin lesion that is seen when hair follicles become inflamed for any reason. Folliculitis is one of the common complications of a hair transplant surgery. Folliculitis usually occurs due to blockage of hair or its sebaceous gland when a newly transplanted follicular unit is healing in its new location. Folliculitis after hair transplantation usually appears as small red or white headed pimples around one, or few, follicular grafts. Folliculitis may present itching, mild pain and minimal discharge. Most cases of folliculitis clear spontaneously in a few days. More aggressive types of folliculitis may need medical or surgical interventions.

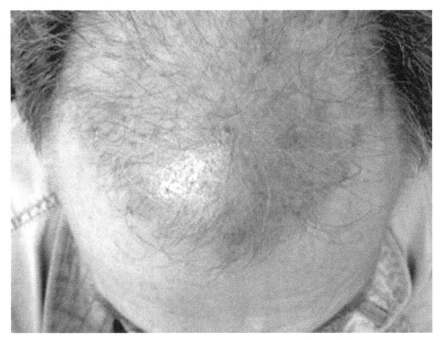

*Folliculitis may be seen a few days to months after a hair transplant surgery. The presence of folliculitis usually does not affect the growth of the transplanted hair.*

Occasionally, the lesions of folliculitis may become painful or their appearance may bother the patient. Simple drainage of the lesions is the only treatment most patients need. A physician's evaluation can best determine whether or not the patient needs antibiotics for the treatment of folliculitis after hair transplant.

## DONOR SCAR

FUE procedure usually does not leave a scar on the donor area. However, strip hair transplant which requires removal of a strip of skin from the donor area, followed by a closing of the wound, generally leaves a linear scar after healing. The strip scar is usually not visible unless a patient decides to shave his head or to keep it very short. There are many procedures that could minimize the appearance of donor scar. One procedure that is performed to minimize the visibility of the scar is trichophytic closure.

Trichophytic closure is when a small wedge is removed along the edge of donor wound before closure. This allows some hair to grow inside the donor wound rather than next to it. Presence of hair follicles in the donor wound minimizes the contrast the scar has with its surrounding areas of the scalp with dense hair. Trichophytic closure could be done on one or both edges of the wound. Doing trichophytic closure on both edges can increase the density of hair that grows inside the scar. This can minimize the visibility of the scar further. Trichophytic closure may result in a donor scar that is almost undetectable in some patients.

The visibility of the donor scar in strip method can be further reduced through a small FUE procedure. In this procedure, the scar is filled with FUE grafts minimizing the contrast of the scar with neighboring areas of the scalp. Transplantation of FUE into the donor scar can be done a few months after the initial surgery once the donor wound is completely healed. Usually, a very small number of FUE grafts are needed to improve the appearance of the scar. This procedure can be completed as a short outpatient procedure.

Other procedures such as medical scalp pigmentation could be used to further minimize the visibility of the donor scar in a patient who requires shaving their head in the future.

Unlike strip procedures, FUE hair transplant does not leave a linear scar. FUE may result in lighter spots or occasionally small pinpoint scars. The scars of FUE may not be visible due to the size or the scattered pattern they have. Some patients may develop hypopigmentation in the areas where the grafts are removed without any obvious scarring. Scalp micropigmentation or medical tattooing can be used to improve the appearance of the FUE donor scars or hypopigmentation if they occur.

## NUMBNESS

Numbness of the scalp could occur after a hair transplant procedure. Numbness could be present in the recipient or donor area. Numbness could happen due to irritation of the sensory nerves of scalp that run under the skin at the donor or recipient area. The initial numbness of anesthetic injections may resolve in a few hours. However, the numbness may occasionally persist for days, or in rare cases weeks, after a hair transplant. No treatment is needed for the numbness and recovery is usually complete in most patients. Injury to some sensory skin nerves may cause permanent numbness in one area of the scalp. This condition is extremely rare and could be avoided in most cases by using the proper technique of surgery.

# HAIR TRANSPLANT FOR OTHER AREAS

## EYEBROW HAIR TRANSPLANT

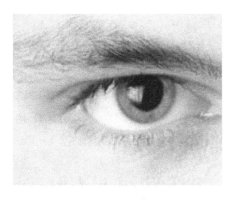

Eyebrow hair transplant is a relatively simple and safe procedure. Eyebrows functionally protect your eyes and are not just a mere cosmetic facial feature. The advance methods of modern hair restoration allow for the creation and restoration of natural looking brows. People who have scars in the brow area, or the ones who have lost the eyebrow hair, are generally very happy to take advantage of an eyebrow hair transplant procedure.

## CAUSES OF EYEBROW HAIR LOSS

The following are often causes of eyebrow hair loss in men and women:

- Congenital inability of growing eyebrow hair. This condition is seen in many members of a family and is easily treated by eyebrow hair transplantation. Some ethnicities may present this type of eyebrow loss more than others.

- Physical trauma such as burns and other accidental injuries.
- Over-plucking or repeated reshaping of eyebrows.
- Continuous damage to the eyebrow follicles in some sports such as boxing.
- Medical disorders such as thyroid diseases.
- Autoimmune disorders such as alopecia areata or lupus.
- Trichotillomania which is an obsessive disorder causing the person to pluck his or her hair obsessively. This could happen to the eyebrow, eyelashes or any other parts of the body that have hair.

A hair transplant can effectively restore partial or total eyebrow loss in various conditions. Hair transplant can only be considered when the underlying medical condition for the hair loss is under control. Hair loss from trichotillomania cannot be performed unless the psychological condition is completely treated and the condition is under control.

## EYEBROW HAIR TRANSPLANT PROCEDURE

Eyebrow transplant is done through harvesting scalp hair from the back of the scalp just like a scalp hair transplant. The removed skin is dissected with microscopic magnification of follicular units. Hair can be harvested with conventional strip techniques or FUE.

After harvesting the donor hair, the recipient area is prepared and small incisions are made in the recipient area. Very tiny incisions produce a tight grip for the follicular unit grafts that are harvested. Angulations of eyebrow hair with sharp angles and their special alignment make eyebrow transplantation more intrinsic than general scalp transplantation. In order to create natural results, and make the eyebrows normal looking, direction and distribution is very important.

The growth of transplanted hair in eyebrows follows the pattern of scalp hair growth. Transplanted eyebrow hairs grow constantly and need to be trimmed more often than normal eyebrow hair. Patients may need up to around 300 follicular unit grafts for each eyebrow depending on the extent of the hair loss area. The number of hair grafts may vary based on the sex and ethnic background of the patient and the individual facial features. Eyebrow hair transplantation is usually performed under local anesthesia and some sedation.

Complications after an eyebrow transplant are minimal. Bruising, swelling and scabbing can be seen during the first few days after an eyebrow transplant. They usually subside 3 to 5 days after the procedure. Daily washings will minimize the amount of scabbing and facilitate healing of implanted hair grafts. Newly transplanted hair to the eyebrow area usually falls out in the first 2 weeks. Patient should be able to see new hair growth from those follicles in about 3 to 6 months. Full results are expected about 6 months from the time of eyebrow transplantation in most people.

## EYELASH HAIR TRANSPLANT

We are often enamored with the eyes of a person. Eyelashes are correlated to beauty in women and men. It is important to note that eyelashes have an anatomical function. They shield the eye from injury. Primarily they are a filter for larger and microscopic particles in the air such as dust and grit. The eye protection afforded by eyelashes is very important.

## CAUSES OF EYELASH LOSS

Eyelash hair loss may be due to many causes. Here is a list of the common causes of eyelash hair loss:

- Industrial accidents resulting in chemical and thermal burns
- Physical trauma due to injuries
- Adverse results from cosmetic enhancements such as eyelid tattoos and traction alopecia associated with long-term use of false eyelashes
- Surgical treatment of injury or tumor that results in removal or eyelash follicles and tissue scarring
- Medical treatments such as radiotherapy or chemotherapy for cancer treatment that results in hair loss
- Trichotillomania which, as described before, is a compulsive hair plucking condition
- Other skin conditions causing hair loss such as alopecia areata or alopecia universalis
- Congenital absence of hair eyelash

## EYELASH TRANSPLANTATION TECHNIQUE

As in all surgical hair transplantation, "living grafts" or hairs follicles are harvested from a donor area or permanent zone (located on the back and sides of the scalp). The transplanted hair will continue to grow in the eyelid the way they would grow in the scalp. The curvature of the transplanted hair is carefully aligned with natural curvature of eyelash hair. Some patients may have to follow a training program for curling the transplanted hair to match the natural curl of their normal eyelashes.

Trimming the hair is always required to maintain the optimum length for the best look and functionality of eyelashes. The preferred method of removal of hair follicles for eyelash transplant is through strip procedure since hair should be kept long. The reason for that is the need to be able to follow the curve of each hair and implant them with the proper angle. The strip removed for an eyelash hair transplant is very small due to the small amount of hair needed.

## MEDICAL TREATMENT FOR EYELASH RESTORATION

Eyelash enhancement has become a popular cosmetic medical treatment. Advancements in understanding the class of drugs known as prostaglandin analogues have led to the rise of this elective medical treatment. Latisse (bimatoprost ophthalmic solution 0.03%) is a relatively new product that has recently gained a lot of popularity. The medication was originally used to treat the increased eyeball pressure in glaucoma. Ophthalmologists noticed stimulated growth and darkening of the patient's eyelashes.

Latisse increases the length of time that hair follicles stay in the growth phase. This helps the eyelashes to grow for longer periods of time and more eyelashes stay in growth phase. This creates longer lashes and more hair density to the eyelashes. Latisse is a great medication for people who want to have thicker fuller eyelashes. This type of medication will not work if the patient has permanently lost their eyelash hair follicles. Eyelash hair transplant is presently the only proven solution for people who have lost their eyelash hair follicles.

# FACIAL AND BODY HAIR TRANSPLANT

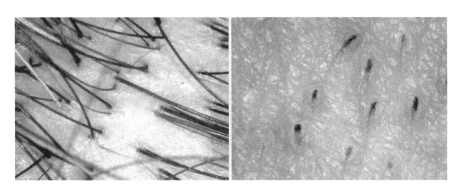

*Comparison of scalp (left) vs. facial (right) hair: Note the difference in density of hair per surface area and the average number of hair in each follicular unit. Scalp hair is denser with more hairs per grafts (over 2hair/graft) while beard hair is less dense with fewer hairs per grafts (1-2 hair/graft)*

## FACIAL TO SCALP HAIR TRANSPLANT

Our hair grows all over our bodies except on the soles of our feet and the palms of our hands, lips and eyelids. Of course, eyelashes are an exception. The utilization of hairs from all over the body for hair transplantation into the scalp has been in practice for many years. Though many men have what appears to be an exceptional supply of donor body hair there is a drawback to extensive use of body hair in hair restoration surgeries.

## BODY HAIR LIFECYCLE

The difference in the life cycle of body hair from different areas of the body makes it one of the last options for scalp hair restoration. Body hair has a long resting phase, and a short growth phase, which means that most of the transplanted hair will stay in the resting phase without having visible hair growth.

On the other hand, facial hair, such as the beard and mustache hair, has a longer growth phase and shorter resting phase. That is why men can grow their facial hair to become really long. Facial hair is also thicker than scalp hair in most people. Thicker hair could be translated as more bulk of hair after hair transplantation. Both longer growth phase and thicker hair shafts make beard hair a better option for scalp hair restoration in comparison to body hair transplant from other areas.

|  | Anagen | Catagen | Telogen |
|---|---|---|---|
| Scalp Hair | 2-6 years | 2-3 weeks | 2-4 months |
| Body Hair | 4-7 months | 3-4 weeks | 9 months |
| Eyebrows | 4-7 months | 3-4 weeks | 9 months |
| Eyelashes | 4-7 weeks | 2-3 weeks | 3-9 weeks |
| Male Facial Hair | 1 year | 2-3 weeks | 7-10 weeks |
| Pubic Hair | 4-8 weeks | 2-3 weeks | 2-3 months |

There are two problems with beard hair restoration. One is

that they are very sparse and removing hair can only be done through FUE procedure. The other problem with using facial hair for scalp transplant is that the facial follicular units have fewer numbers of hairs per unit which means less hair per grafts removed with FUE techniques.

## FACIAL HAIR TRANSPLANTS

Alternately, beard transplants are gaining popularity with the successful advanced techniques of FUE extraction of hair grafts.

People may lose facial hair due to:
- scarring and other scar conditions
- they may not have the ability to grow their mustache or beard genetically
- their natural beard pattern is sparse and/or uneven

In many of these situations, facial hair can be successfully restored with a hair transplant using scalp hair through follicular unit transplantation. We are also able to use some beard hair for transplantation into the mustache area, below the nose and above the upper lip.

In instances where there is a mismatch between the thickness of scalp and beard hair shafts, we use either strip follicular unit transplants or FUE (Follicular Unit Extractions) to harvest hair for mustache hair restoration.

One of the better options for a patient is to use beard hair as the donor source for a FUE procedure. This is most often preferred to avoid facial scarring. The number of needed grafts for the patient is determined by the width of the upper lip and also the shape of mustache that is most proportional with their other facial features.

The cost of facial hair transplantation for mustaches and beards generally follows the same per graft cost as scalp hair transplantation. Results of a mustache hair transplant can be seen as early as 4-6 months following the hair transplant and may continue to improve one year after surgery.

## BODY HAIR TRANSPLANT

Follicular Unit Extraction (FUE) can remove hair from anywhere in the body. FUE procedures are more labor intense and more time consuming so the cost is almost double in comparison to regular strip hair transplant procedures.

Neck hair is not the best option for hair transplantation because those hairs may fall out in older patients. We can use body hair for the hairline, the front or even the crown but you may need multiple surgeries to obtain adequate density in the recipient areas using body hair. As previously noted, body hair has a long resting phase in relation to its growth phase. Therefore, you will have more follicles in resting phase (telogen phase) that do not have any visible hair in comparison to the ones in growth phase (anagen phase) that provide you with actual hair and give you coverage.

Body hair can be considered as an alternative method of hair restoration as long as you, the patient, understands that the end result is not going to be comparable with a scalp hair transplant. This is due to smaller final length of hair and short growth phase (Anagen) as opposed to long resting phase (Telogen) that characterizes body hair. In other words, you may only see a portion of the transplanted hair follicles in growth phase while the remainder stays in resting phase without maintaining a visible hair shaft.

Beard hair transplantation can be a better option. It is generally closer to scalp hair in many patients and has a longer growth phase (which is why it grows to become longer in comparison to body hair). It should be noted that each of these options have pros and cons and patients should be evaluated. It is important that a hair restoration treatment plan is based on the patients' needs and supported by a complete evaluation by a hair transplant surgeon.

# OTHER SCALP SURGERIES

## FACIAL FEMINIZATION SURGERY (FFS)

Hair restoration is helping meet the needs of self-image for many patients. Patients going through the transgender process who may have a full head of hair often desire to have a more feminine hairline. This framing of the face is a large part of their self-image, how they view themselves and how they present themselves to the world.

Hair restoration surgeons are dedicated to taking the advancement of medical science and making them applicable in as many ways as possible for the benefit of their patients. Developing the hairline for transgender patients is meticulous for male to female transgender patients. Many such patients undergo a scalp advancement to move the hairline forward and reduce the depth of the brow typical to male physiognomy.

Today's leading hair transplant surgeons can easily repair the hairline in front of the scar of a transgender patient who has had scalp advancement surgery. It is important not to alter the hairline previously with hair transplant when opting to undergo scalp advancement surgery. If there is less than perfect transplanted hair on the hairline, the hair transplant surgery for feminizing the hairline will be more difficult. This requires removing the hair grafts that are transplanted out of their normal locations and reusing them in the other areas.

## SCAR REVISION

Since the advent of hair restoration surgeries, hair transplant surgeons have been managing and mitigating the challenge of scalp scars from strip hair transplants. Patients may also have a linear scar after undergoing other surgical scalp procedures or neurosurgical operations. Trauma can also be a source of scarring to the head. Although most scars are hidden in patient's native hair, some may become exposed due to their proximity to the hairline or when a patient keeps his hair short.

The size, type and location of scars can determine the techniques available to a surgeon seeking to minimize the appearance of a patient's scar. We have created an algorithm that hair transplant or other cosmetic surgeons can use towards the most effective methods to address scalp scars and the proper surgical or medical approach to them.

A proper physical examination can reveal what proportion of the visibility of scar is due to stretching or hypertrophic reaction and what portion has to do with hair transection.

The scars that are wider than what is expected might have some components of stretching. To improve the visibility of stretched scars, the surgeon needs to use a technique to minimize the contrast between the hairless scar and neighboring areas of the scalp by bringing hair inside the scar.

# HAIR RESTORATION MEDICATION

## EXPECTATIONS FROM MEDICAL HAIR LOSS TREATMENTS

There are many hair loss remedies and products on the market. However, a vast majority of hair loss treatments that are being marketed today are still nothing but "snake oils." A few effective medications for hair loss have been around for over two decades. The development of 5-alpha-reductase inhibitors for treating prostate enlargement marked a landmark breakthrough in hair loss treatment. It is the conversion of the male hormone testosterone to dihydrotestosterone (DHT) that causes health complications in the prostate. As time passes, DHT destroys many hair follicles which is the root cause of male pattern baldness. DHT blockers, along with Rogaine, are the only two types of medications that are FDA-approved for treatment and prevention of patterned baldness.

## 5-ALPHA-REDUCTASE INHIBITORS

There are two powerful medications that were developed for the inhibtion of DHT: finesteride and dutasteride. These two medications were initially used for the treatment of prostate issues such as Benign Prostatic Hyperplasia (BPH). During trials of these 5-alpha-reductase inhibitors, some positive side effect was noted including prevention of hair loss and, in some instances, hair growth. After specific research on hair loss, finasteride (Propecia) garnered FDA approval for the treatment of male pattern baldness. It is now possible to slow down the progression of androgenetic alopecia (male patterned baldness) using finasteride. These discoveries, along with hair transplant advancements, represent the proven answer to hair loss today for many men with typical male pattern baldness. Below is a review of these FDA-approved medications and other treatments that are used to combat hair loss.

## PROPECIA (FINASTERIDE)

Finasteride is the generic name for the brand name medications, Proscar and Propecia. Finasteride was initially produced by MERCK, under the name Proscar, to treat enlarged prostate glands in men. A slightly modified version of Proscar was produced with smaller doses to medically treat hair loss.

In December 1997, the FDA approved a 1mg dose of finasteride for the treatment of androgenetic alopecia or typical male pattern baldness in men. The majority of men who used Propecia have witnessed slower hair loss and even hair growth.

Side effects from finasteride at the 1mg dose are uncommon. In initial studies, the one year drug related side effects were 1.5% greater than in the control group. The data from the research indicated 3.8% sexual dysfunction in men taking finasteride 1mg versus 2.1% in men treated with a placebo.

## HOW FINASTERIDE WORKS

Finasteride specifically inhibits 5-alpha-reductase, the enzyme that converts testosterone into a more potent androgen dihydrotestosterone (DHT). After initial studies on a daily 1 milligram dose of finasteride it was proven that it:

- lowers DHT levels in the scalp significantly when taken on a daily basis
- minimizes the progression of hair loss in the majority of men taking the drug during clinical trials
- promotes a substantial increase of hair growth in trial participants

In the last two decades, most hair restoration doctors have recommended finasteride as the first line of medical hair restoration for men.

## ROGAINE (MINOXIDIL)

Minoxidil was approved prior to Propecia by the FDA for the treatment of male pattern baldness. The pill form of minoxidil, known as 'Linotien', was widely used to treat high blood pressure. Researchers discovered that the people taking the medication were growing hair on the face and other areas of the body.

Researchers came up with the idea that applying topical minoxidil directly on the scalp might grow hair on balding areas. And it did, to varying degrees depending on the extent of the hair loss. This was a revolutionary step in the treatment of hair loss at that time.

Rogaine (minoxidil) has no effect on the hormonal process of hair loss. The positive effects of minoxidil on hair growth usually end with cessation of use. In many cases, patients may even experience the loss of hair that has been kept due to the effect of the medication. This phenomenon is called catch-up hair loss.

Although Rogaine is recognized as an effective treatment for some hair loss sufferers, most doctors do not recommend it as the first line of attack for men suffering from male pattern baldness. The reason behind it is the result of some side by side studies that compared topical minoxidil with oral finasteride. These studies have clearly shown oral finasteride as a more potent option for treatment of male patterned baldness.

## HAIR RESTORATION MEDICATION SIDE EFFECTS

Minoxidil and finasteride are the two FDA-approved medications for hair restoration. Millions of people now choose this medical treatment to effectively reduce hair loss. In addition, finasteride (Propecia) is prescribed in our advanced technology Parsa Mohebi Hair Restoration centers throughout Los Angeles. Finasteride is very effective pre, and post, hair transplant surgery. It does not matter which form of follicular unit transplant (FUT) a patient is electing to undergo. It is effective whether one is having a 'Strip Method' surgery or FUE hair transplant.

As with any medication, it is important to understand the possible side effects (no matter how rare). As finasteride is a successful and strategic hair restoration medical treatment that we employ in our centers, it is important to clarify the possible risks or side effects of this treatment.

## FINASTERIDE (PROPECIA)

The side effects from this treatment are not as common as 'urban legends' would have people to believe. Studies show that when a patient uses the most often prescribed 1 mg dose, the reported side effects were usually reversible. In fact, it is important to note that, after a one year study of the drug, related side effects were much greater than the placebo control group. Finasteride side effects were only 1.5% greater in the group taking the medication.

Sexual dysfunction was the reported side effect by men in the control group. During the study, the percentage of men in the control group with that complaint was only 3.8%. This is compared to 2.1% of men with the same complaint in the placebo group during the year long study. In addition, a 5 year side effects profile yielded the following statistics: decreased libido reported in 0.3%, erectile dysfunction reported at 0.3% and decreased volume of ejaculate at 0.0%.

## SEXUAL DYSFUNCTION

The general word out there is that impotence is a common side effect in men taking finasteride. However, the scientific data does not report it to the degree of severity that we often hear about from patients in our clinics.

Based on the research data reports, sexual dysfunction occurs at the onset of the medical treatment. In some instances, it is reported later. It is important to note that within a few weeks after cessation of the treatment, the sexual dysfunction side effects were reversed. Nearly sixty percent of all men staying on treatment noted that the side effects subsided.

Although the company Merck has added the possibility of irreversible side effects of Propecia, the idea that sexual dysfunction continues after stopping the medication has yet to be substantiated in studies and these reports need to be confirmed with well-designed medical research.

## LONG-TERM BENEFITS AND RISKS

The benefits of finasteride are strictly to scalp hair which is thinning or undergoing miniaturization. Finasteride does not restore fully miniaturized hair follicles. This means that if baldness is complete, it will not work. Thinning scalp hair or miniaturizing hair is halted and other scalp hair does not begin the process of miniaturization. This means it is not effective for people who are completely bald. The primary benefit of finasteride is to slow down or stop hair loss from male pattern baldness.

Best results are reported for the first year of use and a modest decrease in second year of use. Long term benefits are still unknown but men who have taken finasteride for five years report that it still works.

# OTHER HAIR LOSS TREATMENTS FOR WOMEN

The most common type of hair loss in women in which patients have significant thinning or miniaturization of hair throughout the scalp is known as Female Patterned Baldness (FPB). Female patterned baldness is generally characterized with diffuse hair loss. Women who have diffuse miniaturization (fineness of scalp hair) may be good candidates for medical treatment with minoxidil (Rogaine).

Women with more advanced hair loss may not respond to the medical treatment. Some women with non-diffused hair loss who have preserved hair quality on some areas of their scalp can be good candidates for hair transplant surgery. Many of these women may be suffering from male patterned hair loss in which they preserve the quality of hair on the back and side of scalp while losing it in other areas.

Many women may lose their scalp hair due to other medical conditions that also may present with diffuse hair loss. Diagnosis of this type of hair loss could be made with laboratory work or scalp biopsy in most of these women. Depending on the type of hair loss, a hair loss specialist may elect one or a combination of these options.

| Diagnosis | MPB (local balding) | FPB (Diffused thining) | Other medical conditions |
|---|---|---|---|
| Treatment | Hair transplant anti-androgen - if hyperandro-genism exists | Rogaine Cosmetic change | Treat underly-ing condition |

Table 1: Association of each diagnosis of female patterned hair loss with its treatment options

In addition to medical and surgical treatments, an experienced hair specialist can cosmetically help women through cosmetic changes. The proper use of cosmetic products and hair styling should be part of most hair loss consultations. A hair specialist may also review the options for hairstyle for maximum coverage and to hide the thinning areas of the scalp. At times when the hair loss is very advanced, and the patients are not candidates for medical or surgical treatments of hair loss, wigs or synthetic hair systems may be the last solution.

## CONCEALERS FOR HAIR LOSS

There are two popular keratinized fiber products used to create the illusion of thickness for thinning hair and early baldness. Microfibers such as Toppik and Caboki are used by many women in different stages of hair loss. These products are sprinkled into the thinning area and worked through into the hairstyle creating the illusion of more hair. The idea is that the small microfiber can attach itself to the hair shaft and make hair look thicker as well as coloring the scalp to minimize the contrast between the hair color and skin tone. The drawback is that these products can come off on clothes and furniture when touched. Similarly, there are sprays to minimize the contrast between the scalp and hair color by painting the scalp surface.

## FOUNDATIONS OR COVER UPS

Foundation products like those used on the face are sometimes used on the scalp. Foundations are used when there is not much visible hair in one area like men who only have a blading spot on the crown area. An example of those products is DermMatch that can be used by people who suffer from the appearance of a balding patch on their scalp. By choosing a color close to the individual's hair color, minor thinning or baldness can be blended with a cover up. Like microfibers and sprays, these products can come off after use.

## LASER FOR HAIR LOSS TREATMENT

Research on laser treatments for hair loss is not yet definitive enough for many hair restoration doctors to justify its use. These devices are currently available without a standardization of form and functionality. Here are some of the available options for hair loss treatment:

- Laser comb
- Laser hood
- Laser hat

There has been anecdotal information on the effectiveness of some of these devices. Those are mostly the ones with adequate amount of laser beam. People with diffuse hair loss, like many women with female patterned hair loss, seem to benefit best from it. The laser cap treats the entire scalp with 224 individual red 5mw – 650 laser diodes and some hair loss specialists and their patients report positive results. Despite the reports on their effectiveness in some patients, more research is needed before any of the laser devices find their place as an effective hair loss treatment.

# ADVANCEMENT IN HAIR RESTO-RATION TECHNOLOGIES

## MEGASESSION AND GIGASESSION HAIR TRANSPLANTS

In addition to the increase in the quality of the hair transplants, there has been a high demand for transplant procedures with a larger number of grafts. Megasession hair transplants (over 2000 grafts) or gigasessions transplants (grafts over 3500) are new advancements in hair transplantation. In these procedures, a surgeon can restore a large balding area in only one session. The time involved in each hair transplantation, combined with the long waiting period to see the full results, makes multiple surgeries unattractive to patients. Mega and giga sessions can eliminate the need for additional surgeries in most cases.

Of course, hair transplants with large number of grafts require special techniques and skills. A more efficient surgical team is also required for those procedures. Many factors should be considered during a large hair transplant procedure. Minimizing the time that hair follicles must stay out of body is vital in larger procedures. Introduction of simultaneous extraction and placement and sequential strip removal (Parsa Mohebi 2010) in which the strip is removed in two sections rather than one can reduce the time grafts stay out of body by half. Both simultaneous extraction and placement and sequential strip removal can increase the survival of the grafts by minimizing the time they spend out of body.

Calculating the maximum safe number of grafts is one of the crucial elements in strip procedures. This calculation has been facilitated using the Laxometer (Parsa Mohebi 2007) which measures the free mobility of the scalp so the surgeon knows how much of the scalp skin is safe to remove.

## LAXOMETER

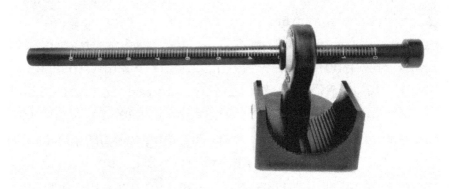

A laxometer is a device invented and developed by Dr. Parsa Mohebi for measuring scalp laxity more precisely. Scalp laxity is a crucial factor in most hair transplant procedures which are performed with the removal of a donor strip from the permanent zone at the back of the head. These donor hairs are genetically resistant to the adverse effects of DHT on hair follicles. Hair transplant surgeons used to measure the laxity of the scalp manually. The surgeons often recorded the mobility of the scalp before hair transplants with terms such as loose, moderate and severe tightness. Manual measurement of the scalp laxity was an approximate gauge and was not always accurate.

The Laxometer is a measuring device that is used to calculate the laxity of the scalp. An accurate measurement of scalp laxity is critical when determining how wide the donor strip can be. This breakthrough in hair transplant technology allows surgeons to determine a precise measurement. In the case of a less desirable scalp laxity, the number can be verifiably increased as a result of patients doing daily scalp exercises. The patient's improved scalp laxity allows for the removing of a larger strip of scalp increasing the number of FUs available for hair transplantation.

## MOTORIZED FUE TRANSPLANTS

In the last few years, we have been witnessing the emergence of several motorized FUE devices. These devices were developed to solve the following issues with FUE procedures:
- high transection rate
- slow speed of grafts extraction
- the trauma on scalp tissue

Independent comparison studies to ascertain the success levels of these devices in resolving these issues have been minimal. Presently, hair restoration surgeons adopt one or a few of these methods to provide their patients with the best results.

## FUE TRANSPLANT WITH NEW SYSTEMS

The advanced improvements in modern hair transplantation techniques provide better results for hair restoration patients. Follicular Unit Extraction (FUE) traditionally has been done through punching out hair grafts manually. In this procedure, a very small punch device assists the surgeon in removing the follicular units from the donor area. The manual removal of the follicular units could be time consuming and, at times, provide low quality grafts. The newer and more modern techniques of hair restoration provide a variety of motorized devices that help the surgeon remove grafts at a higher speed and better quality. Several different motorized devices are available on the market. Some of the motorized devices that are used to harvest follicular units are SAFE System, NeoGraft, Cole System and Trivellini FUE Device.

We have performed several experiments on different motorized and manual techniques of Follicular Unit Extraction (FUE) in our Los Angeles hair transplant center since 2010. The result of our study has helped us chose more efficient devices and punches that guarantee the best outcome for our patients. Our new systems can help minimize the risk of damage to the follicular grafts while they can be harvested at a reasonable speed.

## ROBOTIC FUE HAIR RESTORATION

The Robotic System (ARTAS) is one of the most advanced techniques in FUE hair restoration. ARTAS has a robotic arm that allows for harvesting hair from the donor area in patients with male patterned baldness using the Follicular Unit Extraction method (r-FUE).

ARTAS uses computer assistance to harvest hair follicles for hair transplantation. The system incorporates several elements in its operation including an image guided robotic arm and special imaging software that coordinate together for harvesting follicular unit grafts both individually and precisely. The ARTAS System enables our medical staff to extract hair follicular units more rapidly and with higher precision.

The system is equipped with a sophisticated algorithm that facilitates mapping and collecting of follicular units. Random harvesting of the units is designed by the system to minimize the risk of scarring and over-harvesting. Patients who receive the ARTAS FUE procedure can usually return to normal activities the day after the procedure like the other types of FUE procedures.

## How does it Work?

The hair transplant surgeon determines and marks the donor area, also known as permanent zone, on the back and sides of the scalp. After application of the numbing medications, the patient is placed in a sitting position while putting their face over a donut shaped pillow for maximum stability and comfort. Then, a tensioner is placed over the donor area to stabilize the skin for the harvesting process. ARTAS uses several cameras to capture microscopic video images of the patient's follicular units. The hairs are then easily identified by the 3D microscopic camera of the robot.

Hair direction and exit angles are not the same in different parts of the scalp. The robot constantly monitors the exit angle of hair and calculates the internal hair axis based on the collected data. The ARTAS software identifies and computes hair features such as number of hair per follicular unit, hair exit angle, direction and overall density of hair in each area. The gathered information is processed with ARTAS's algorithm and generates a plan for harvesting hair follicles with high accuracy.

The robotic arm will be adjusted based on the processed information from the 3D camera system. After identification of individual follicular units, they will be reaped individually with the robotic dual punch system while optimizing the quality of the extracted hair follicles. The doctor and medical staff operate the system by making adjustments to fine tune the dissection of follicular unit grafts.

The ARTAS robotic hair harvesting system is an advanced device that enhances the safety and precision of hair restoration procedures. Combination of our artistic approach, and robotic advanced technology, makes r-FUE a safe and effective hair restoration method.

Robotic hair restoration has its own limitations and cannot extract hair from other parts of the body or certain areas of scalp. It is best to leave the decision of what instrument to use for your hair transplant surgery to your surgeon.

## STEM CELL AND HAIR MULTIPLICATION

Hair multiplication or hair cloning is a method of multiplying hair follicles and generating a larger number of donor hairs for transplantation purposes. The growth and development of hair follicles is regulated by two types of stem cells residing in each hair follicle. Those are the Dermal Papilla and the Bulge area stem cells. Scientists have been attempting to replicate hair cells and create more hair for transplantation purposes in and out of the body.

Although the initial studies show the success of hair multiplications in the lab, the research for hair multiplication has been progressing very slowly due to many factors:

1. Hair loss has a detrimental effect on patients' lives. However, it has not yet been recognized as a crucial medical problem in order to warrant more funding for hair loss research.

2. Hair multiplication studies are usually done in private settings without the support of larger medical institutions such as universities and NIH (National Institute of Health).

3. The duplication time for hair stem cell is extremely slow in cell cultures. This makes the overall period of hair cell duplication timelier which adds exponentially to the duration and cost of most hair stem cell studies.

The stem cell studies for multiplying hair should go through different phases. The last necessary phase in the development of every new medical treatment is 'clinical trials'. This phase is done on volunteer patients with long-term follow-up. This is to evaluate the risk of long-term complications associated with the treatment. We are not aware of any hair cloning study that has reached the clinical trials. This makes it unlikely to have any hair cloning procedures available to the public in the next few years.

# GENE THERAPY: A NEW FRONTIER IN HAIR RESTORATION

Gene therapy is still in its infancy. To date, there are only a few examples of gene therapy success in the treatment of alopecia. Still, gene therapy represents the newest frontier in medical hair restoration treatment.

Gene therapy could be one of the most perfect techniques for solving patterned baldness. It is the process of altering cell function by changing genes that are responsible for unwanted traits. Gene therapy requires learning how an inherited medical condition occurs at the DNA molecular level. Hair follicles with DHT-sensitive cells could be changed into follicles with DHT-resistant cells with gene therapy. This makes it possible for the hair follicles to continue growing new hairs for a lifetime.

Gene therapy involves several very difficult steps to achieve a viable medical treatment for baldness.

1. The first step is to determine which genes among the tens of thousands of genes on strands of DNA are involved in the characteristic for hereditary alopecia.

2. The next step will be to figure out how to alter the targeted genes to give instructions for making the slightly different proteins that will achieve the desired effect.

3. The final step is getting the target cells in the patient to incorporate the new and improved genes as replacements for the old undesirable genes.

# GROWTH FACTORS FOR HAIR GROWTH

Growth factors are important in the process of hair growth. We need to identify the necessary growth factors in the process of hair loss in order to be able to control the process. We know that the lack of some growth factors is responsible for hair loss in men and women. This means that we should be able to modulate the hair development system by manipulating the levels of growth factors.

# PLATELET RICH PLASMA (PRP)

Utilizing PRP, or Platelet Rich Plasma, for hair restoration is a concept that was developed based on the effects growth factors could have on the growth of human hair.

More studies are necessary to identify the effective timing for growth factors to be used for hair restoration or to slow down the process of hair loss.

Platelet Rich Plasma (PRP) has been hinted at, and suggested, as a possible treatment for hair loss. Using growth factors as a means of restoring hair, as well as preventing hair loss, has been an ongoing project in the field of hair restoration. The PRP that is extracted from the patient's own blood contains proteins such as growth factors and is used as a potential hair restoration treatment by some centers.

# PRP AND HAIR GROWTH EXPLAINED

PRP is extracted from the non-cellular component of blood. PRP includes platelets and growth factors. The plasma extracted from a patient's blood in an outpatient setting contains growth factors such as:

- Platelet-Derived Growth Factor (PDGF)
- Transforming Growth-Factor-Beta (TGF-b)
- Vascular Endothelial Growth Factor (VEGF)
- Epidermal Growth Factor (EGF)
- Fibroblast Growth Factor-2 (FGF-2)
- Insulin Like Growth Factor – (IGF)

These growth factors help with several stages of healing after a patient suffers from injuries or inflammatory conditions.

The presence of the above factors is the reason PRP injections have been linked to treating a variety of medical conditions by promoting tissue and organ healing as well as soft tissue inflammation tendon/fascia/muscle injuries. Since some of these growth factors are also involved in the growth of hair, it has been assumed that PRP could be used as an option to treat baldness.

## PRP PREPARATION

Harvesting PRP is actually a simple process that involves collecting blood from a patient and separating the plasma from it by spinning it in a centrifuge device. The separation process splits the cellular elements inside the blood, such as the RBCs (Red Blood Cells) and WBCs (White Blood Cells), from the plasma (liquid) part of the blood that has growth factors and platelets.

Most studies on PRP were done on a small number of patients

with inconsistent results. Many clinicians use PRP by itself as regular injections to the scalp and some use it in conjunction with other hair loss treatments such as hair transplants or medical treatments. The early studies on PRP were not substantiated enough to introduce PRP as an effective treatment of hair loss with long lasting results.

At Johns Hopkins Medical School, we were able to conduct a number of studies using growth factors for wound healing. The issue with using the growth factors for wound healing and other purposes is that these proteins are very labile and are removed from the tissue in just a few minutes. A continuous source of growth factors is needed in order to see any stimulating results on a cellular level that can support a sustaining growth. Our focus of studies at Johns Hopkins wound healing lab was to provide a more continuous source for growth factors that were needed to help wound healing. We have been able to do that in experimental levels through injecting the genes responsible for production of those growth factors to the skin cells. Creating such a mechanism in balding skin seems to be a more promising means of using growth factors for hair growth as well as for wound healing in the future.

## NEW MEDICATIONS FOR HAIR RESTORATION

Medications that are presently approved to combat hair loss are Rogaine (minoxidil) and Propecia (finasteride). These medications counteract androgenic alopecia or genetic patterned hair loss. Both these medications require ongoing use for the best results. Both finasteride and minoxidil can slow down the process of hair loss but they are limited and may not be able to restore someone's hair to its full density in the long run. The result is significantly expensive over time and also poses a risk of some adverse reaction from long-term use.

As doctors and scientists improve their body of knowledge on how the hair cycle works and how it is controlled metabolically and genetically, they will be able to discover more effective products that help hair loss sufferers.

A current medication on the market, Dutasteride is prescribed to treat benign enlarged prostate glands and could also be used for hair loss soon. Dutasteride is proven to be more effective than Propecia. Dutasteride is also prescribed under the brand name Avodart.

Dutasteride is a 5-alpha-reductase inhibitor that is taken as a pill. Dutasteride has been shown to dramatically reduce the levels of DHT by blocking the conversion of testosterone. Elevated levels of DHT can also cause enlarged prostate glands in men over time.

Narrowing targeting, while reducing side effects, is the next level in increasing the overall effectiveness and desirability of hair loss medications. The future could also hold the opportunity to develop topical lotions for scalp application that more effectively block the DHT.

In the future we will be able to better affect the DHT levels in the cells in the hair follicles. This may result in better control of hair loss and can reduce unwanted side effects of these medications. It is highly possible that medications of the future will be combined with shampoos or hair conditioners and these products will become a common way to keep hair loss at a minimum.

It is clear the future of hair loss treatment holds great promise from new medications, the advances in hair cloning and gene therapy. These treatments are years, or maybe decades, away from FDA approval and before they are available for practical treatments.

The great news is that today's treatment methods, including drugs such as Propecia, and surgical procedures such as Follicular Unit Transplantation (FUT), are available now to provide natural and permanent solutions for hair loss. These methods are sufficient for many men and women to restore and maintain a full head of hair without the need to undergo any other treatments.

# OTHER SCALP PROCEDURES

## SCAR REVISION

Going bald negatively impacts a person's self-image and esteem. The effects of scalp scars are likewise adverse on a person's well-being. One of the most rewarding aspects in hair restoration is the positive impact that a successful hair transplant has on the happiness of patients. Scar revision also has this type of profound effect on many people who suffer from unwanted scalp scars.

First and foremost, we believe in prevention. A properly selected wound closure technique and utilization of proper instruments can make a difference in the final appearance of a scalp scar. In some instances, scar development is inevitable and the surgeon needs to know how to manage a scar to reduce the visibility of scalp scars. Based on the type of scar we recommend several methods of scar revision:

*Simple Scar Revision*
Due to technical or congenital issues, the donor scar can become wide as it heals. The scar can be provisioned with a simple minor surgery. A simple scar revision is performed by the surgeon removing the old scar followed by closing the wound edges with the proper technique in one or two layers.

*Scar Revision and Trichophytic Closure*
The surgeon removes the scar and closes the wound in a manner which allows hair to grow inside the scar. The eventual growth of hair minimizes the contrast between scar and surrounding areas of the scalp.

*FUE Transplant*
Utilizing follicular unit extraction (FUE), we are able to take a small number of donor hairs (as needed) from the permanent zone of scalp. The harvested follicular unit grafts are carefully implanted inside the scar. Since FUE is the individual removal of hair units, there will be minimal to no scarring in the areas where grafts are removed. The newly transplanted hair blends the scar making it almost undetectable in most cases. Some people may need more than one surgery for the optimum result.

*SMP (Scalp-Micro Pigmentation)*
In this procedure, fine needles are used to insert dermal pigments in the skin to create the illusion of stubble hair within the scar. The pigments are chosen to emulate the color of the person's hair. This non-surgical method of scar revision reduces the visibility of scars.

## SCALP REDUCTION

Scalp reduction was once a common choice among hair loss procedures. The availability of follicular unit transplantation with undetectable results had made scalp reduction obsolete. Today's leading hair restoration centers utilize advanced technology and sophisticated techniques that produce more natural and undetectable results. There are perhaps some rare exceptions when this procedure could be an alternative such as burn scars or congenital scalp lesions.

This surgery was initially described in 1977 by Drs. Blanchard and Blanchard. Scalp reduction reduces the size of the bald area by excising a substantial portion of bald scalp and suturing. Drs. Martin Unger and Walter Unger recommended a combination of scalp reduction and modern hair transplant. They believed the use of these procedures improved their overall results for hair restoration. Scalp laxity is very critical to the success of scalp reduction and, for the same reason, it is not a good solution for many people who do not have adequate scalp laxity.

## SCALP MICROPIGMENTATION (SMP)

Scalp Micropigmentation (SMP), also known as trichopigmentation, is a revolutionary new cosmetic procedure performed at Parsa Mohebi Hair Restoration to improve the aesthetic appearance of a patient's scalp using dermal pigments. SMP can imitate the look of a close shaved head or blend in with the patients' natural hair when the appearance of more fullness is desired. The procedure is relatively non-invasive and is usually performed without anesthesia.

## WHO IS A GOOD CANDIDATE FOR SMP?

Ideal candidates for SMP are people who do not have adequate hair to cover their entire balding area with the density they desire. Patients with scalp scar due to old methods of hair transplant or other procedures can minimize the visibility of the scar as well. The most common applications of SMP are for the following groups:

**Scalp Visibility after Hair Transplant:** Men or women who had a hair transplant in the past but still have some scalp visibility due to thinner hair and a large area of baldness. This condition is known as donor/recipient mismatch. Donor/recipient mismatch is when the amount, or volume, of donor hair a patient has cannot provide adequate coverage for the entire balding area.

**Female Hair Loss:** Women who have typical female patterned baldness and are not good candidates for a hair transplant. These patients don't have sufficient permanent hair anywhere in the scalp that can be transplanted. Most of these women are dependent on either microfiber like Toppik or a hair system. SMP can minimize the contrast between their hair and scalp and create the illusion of fullness.

**Shaved Head:** For men with male patterned baldness that decide to shave their head and don't want the typical balding horseshoe pattern to be visible. SMP can create the appearance of a full head of hair in these men. SMP can create the appearance of short hair stubbles that mimic a full head of hair.

**Scalp Scar:** Men or women with scalp scars due to trauma, surgery or a previous strip hair transplant that are now planning to shave their head and want to get rid of the visibility of the scars.

**Other Types of Hair Loss:** Anyone with any type of hair loss who want to improve the appearance of the balding area. Examples are skin conditions such as Alopecia Capitis, Alopecia Areata in the head and face, Alopecia Cicatricial or post radiation hair loss.

SMP can create a close shaved look in patients where the patterned baldness at the front and crown is noticeable by using dermal pigments matched to the patients' hair color. The procedure can also produce the look of more hair density in patients who have thinning hair by minimizing the visibility of the scalp. This eliminates the need for microfiber products such as Toppik which, while effective in filling out one's hair, are messy and come off easily.

**Benefits of Scalp Micropigmentation**

Here are more benefits of scalp micropigmentation:
- Increases the appearance of density and thickness of thinning hair
- Simulates the look of a closely shaved head for completely bald patients
- Helps conceal scars of previous scalp procedures such as donor scars in former hair transplant patients
- Improves the look of hair density in men and women suffering from patterned hair loss
- Effective treatment for patients suffering from conditions where hair transplant cannot be a good solution such as Alopecia Areata, Alopecia Totalis and Alopecia Universalis
- Effective treatment for hypopigmentation that may be seen after FUE procedures on the donor area

# APPENDIX

## PATIENT 1

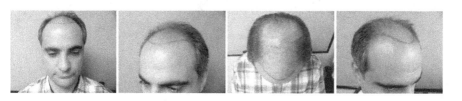

*Class VI hair loss. 12 months elapsed after a hair transplant with 3288 grafts.*

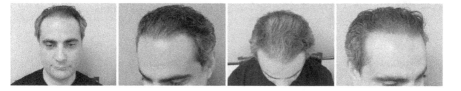

## PATIENT 2

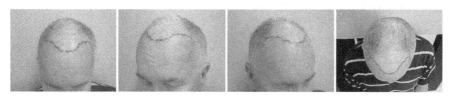

*Class IV hair loss. 6 months elapsed after a hair transplant with 2544 grafts.*

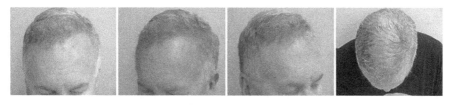

## PATIENT 3

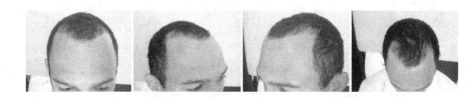

*Class III hair loss. 12 months elapsed after a hair transplant with 1326 grafts.*

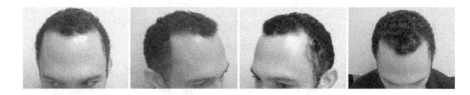

## PATIENT 4

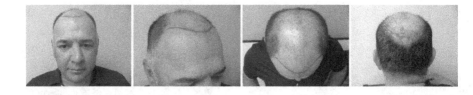

*Class VII hair loss. 12 months elapsed after a hair transplant with 3702 grafts.*

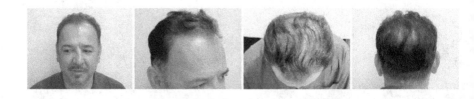

## PATIENT 5

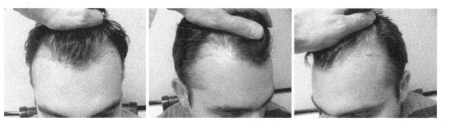

*Class III hair loss. 12 months elapsed after a hair transplant with 1570 grafts.*

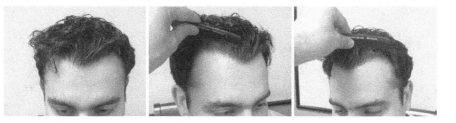

## PATIENT 6

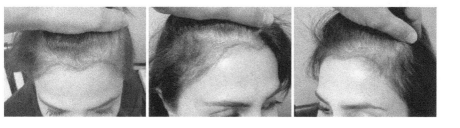

*Class III hair loss. 12 months elapsed after a hair transplant with 1570 grafts.*

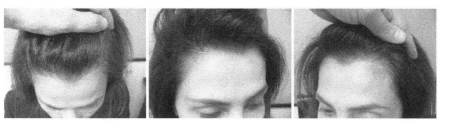

## PATIENT 7

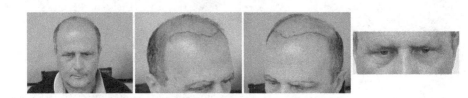

*Class VI hair loss. 6 months elapsed after a hair transplant with 3251 grafts..*

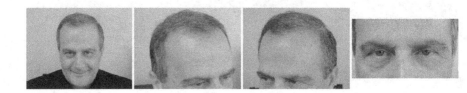

## PATIENT 8

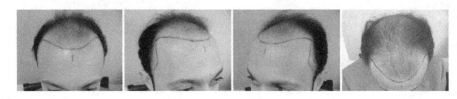

*Class VI hair loss. 10 months elapsed after a hair transplant with 4573 grafts.*

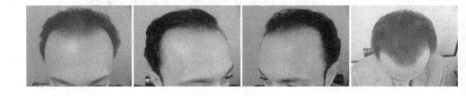

# Parsa Mohebi, MD

## PATIENT 9

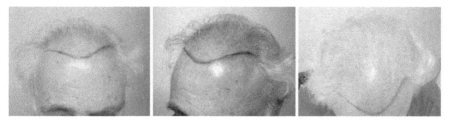

*Class VII hair loss. 10 months elapsed after a hair transplant with 2805 grafts.*

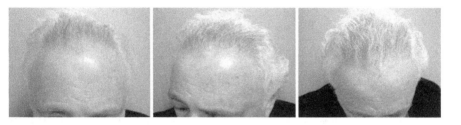

## PATIENT 10

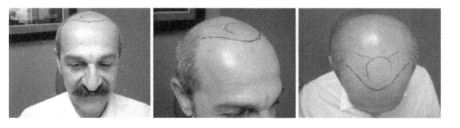

*Class VII hair loss. 10 months elapsed after second hair transplant with total of 5612 grafts.*

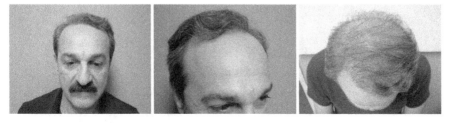

## PATIENT 11

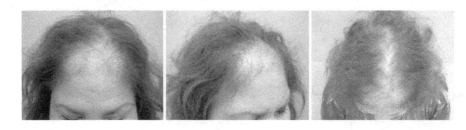

*Class FPH hair loss. 6 months elapsed after second hair transplant with total of 4740 grafts.*

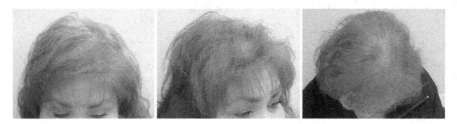

## PATIENT 12

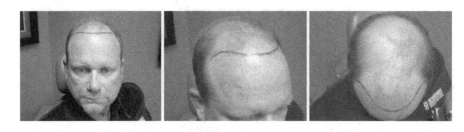

*Class FPH hair loss. 6 months elapsed after second hair transplant with total of 4740 grafts.*

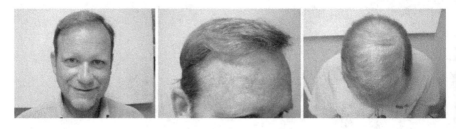

## PATIENT 13

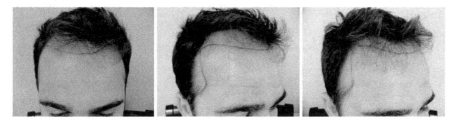

*Class III hair loss. 10 months elapsed after a hair transplant with 2298 grafts.*

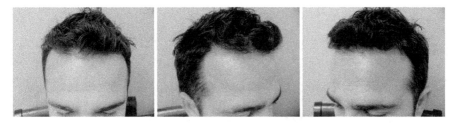

## PATIENT 14

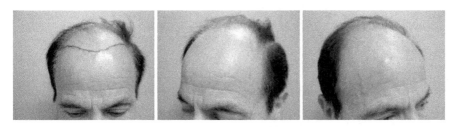

*Class VI hair loss. 12 months elapsed after a hair transplant with 3114 grafts.*

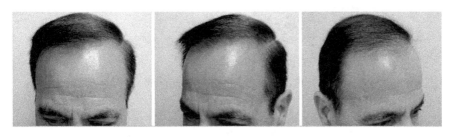

## PATIENT 15

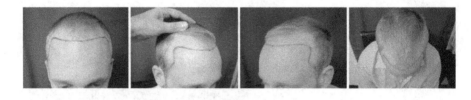

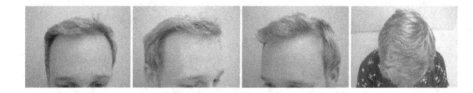

*Class III hair loss. 10 months elapsed after a hair transplant with 2439 grafts.*

## PATIENT 16

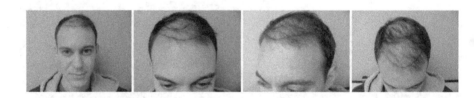

*Top Thinning hair loss. 12 months elapsed after a hair transplant with 3477 grafts.*

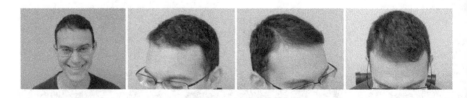

# INDEX

**I**

immune disorder 48
immune system 13
implantation 59
increase blood flow 25
infection 40, 48
inherit 66
Internal Revenue Service 3
iron deficiency 16, 66

**K**

keratin 28
keratinized protein 3, 10
keratinized 123

**L**

lab work 46
laser treatments 124
Latisse 106
laxometer 24, 127, 128
licensed professional 15
local anesthesia 104
local hair loss 38, 47, 48
lupus 48, 67, 103

**M**

macro 46, 85
magnification 45, 56, 59, 103
male and female pattern hair loss 30
male hormone 33, 67, 116
male hormones 23, 29, 49
male or female 15, 31, 39, 42, 93

male pattern baldness 11, 16, 18, 30, 34, 35, 43, 64, 116, 117, 118, 119, 121
male patterned 4, 5, 18, 21, 25, 32, 34, 42, 50, 68, 117, 119, 122, 129, 142
male patterned hair loss 18, 50, 122
male pattern hair loss 45
manual methods 75
mechanism 34, 75, 136
medical condition 10, 46, 78, 103, 133
medical evaluation 11, 43, 65
medical hair restoration 30, 53, 118
medical problems 44, 66, 78
medical professionals 33
medical technicians 58
medical treatments 27, 47, 105, 136
medulla 29
mega and giga sessions 126
megasession hair transplants 126
memory recall 6
Merck 117, 121
micro-evaluation 45
microfibers 123, 124
microscopic 21, 27, 42, 45, 46, 49, 63, 66, 67, 68, 103, 105, 130
microscopic evaluation 21, 27, 42,

| | | | | |
|---|---|---|---|---|
| permanent hair loss | *14, 19, 20, 21, 25, 30* | recipient sites | *59, 69, 95* |
| permanents | *15* | remedies | *54, 116* |
| permanent zone | *47, 58, 67, 68, 105, 127, 130, 140* | remedy | *9* |
| physical evaluation | *47* | replacement techniques | *56* |
| pigmentation | *62, 100, 140* | Robotic Hair Restoration | *75, 76, 131* |
| Platelet Rich Plasma | *134, 135, 136* | robotic system | *129* |
| poor circulation | *21, 22* | Rogaine | *26, 36, 47, 49, 116, 118, 119, 122, 136* |
| positive impact | *7, 139* | Roman Empire | *53* |
| Professor Dom Unger | *53* | | |
| progesterone | *12, 67* | | |
| progesterone levels | *12, 67* | | |
| prolactin | *46* | | |
| Propecia | *26, 37, 39, 49, 97, 117, 118, 119, 121, 136, 137, 138* | | |
| Proscar | *117* | | |
| prostaglandin | *106* | | |
| protein | *3, 10, 28, 57* | | |
| psychological disorder | *38* | | |
| psychological effects | *63* | | |
| psychological impact | *4, 5* | | |
| psychological impacts | *4, 5* | | |
| psychological variables | *4, 5* | | |
| punch grafts | *55* | | |

## R

| | | | |
|---|---|---|---|
| radiation therapy | *38* | | |
| recipient areas | *56, 58, 86, 111* | | |
| recipient dominance | *55* | | |

## S

| | |
|---|---|
| SAFE System | *129* |
| satisfaction | *5, 47* |
| scalp | *13, 15, 18, 19, 20, 22, 23, 24, 25, 30, 35, 36, 37, 39, 40, 41, 42, 43, 45, 46, 47, 49, 53, 54, 57, 58, 63, 66, 67, 68, 71, 72, 75, 77, 79, 80, 83, 86, 87, 92, 93, 97, 99, 100, 101, 103, 104, 105, 108, 109, 110, 111, 112, 113, 114, 115, 118, 121, 122, 123, 124, 125, 127, 128, 130, 131, 136, 137, 139, 140, 141, 142, 143* |
| scalp advancement | *113, 114* |
| scalp circulation | *22* |
| scalp examination | *45* |

CPSIA information can be obtained
at www.ICGtesting.com
Printed in the USA
LVHW05s1635241018
594669LV00009B/696/P